The Incense Bible
Plant Scents That Transcend World Culture, Medicine, and Spirituality

The Incense Bible
Plant Scents That Transcend World Culture, Medicine, and Spirituality

Kerry Hughes, MSc

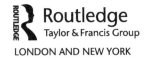

Routledge
Taylor & Francis Group

LONDON AND NEW YORK

First published 2007 by The Haworth Press, Inc.

This edition published 2014 by Routledge
711 Third Avenue, New York, NY 10017 USA
2 Park Square, Milton Park, Abingdon, Oxon OX14 4RN

Routledge is an imprint of the Taylor & Francis Group, an informa business

PUBLISHER'S NOTE
The development, preparation, and publication of this work has been undertaken with great care. However, the Publisher, employees, editors, and agents of The Haworth Press are not responsible for any errors contained herein or for consequences that may ensue from use of materials or information contained in this work. The Haworth Press is committed to the dissemination of ideas and information according to the highest standards of intellectual freedom and the free exchange of ideas. Statements made and opinions expressed in this publication do not necessarily reflect the views of the Publisher, Directors, management, or staff of The Haworth Press, Inc., or an endorsement by them.

Cover design by Marylouise E. Doyle.

Library of Congress Cataloging-in-Publication Data

Hughes, Kerry.
   The incense bible : plant scents that transcend world culture, medicine, and spirituality / Kerry Hughes.
      p. cm.
   Includes bibliographical references.
   ISBN: 978-0-7890-2169-4 (hard : alk. paper)
   ISBN: 978-0-7890-2170-0 (soft : alk. paper)
      1. Incense. I. Title.
GT3031.H84 2007
585'.4—dc22

                                                                    2006034708

ISBN 978-1-315-86478-5 (eISBN)

In precious memory of Chief Phil Crazybull, 1949-2006. I will take the time to light the white sage in your honor, and with gratitude for your teachings. May your teachings live on and reach the children of the world. *Mitakuye Oyasin.*

Dedicated to my mom and dad, Ethel and Gary Hughes, and my grandmother, Mary Howorth, for all their love and support through the years. Blessings to my brother and sister, Owen and Holly.

ABOUT THE AUTHOR

Kerry Hughes, MSc, is an ethnobotanist who specializes in product development, plant commercialization, agricultural development, and medical writing for the natural products industry. She is the founder of EthnoPharm Consulting and the EthnoPharm Botanical Database™ and has worked with natural product companies throughout the United States and in South America, Europe, and Asia, involving the development of plant products for the functional food, dietary supplement, specialty food, and cosmetic markets. She writes and speaks frequently on the subject of botanicals, their use in medicine and science, and the development of botanical products from indigenous cultures, and is co-author of *Botanical Medicines: The Desk Reference for Major Herbal Supplements, Second Edition* (Haworth).

CONTENTS

Preface

This book is intended to represent "multiple dips in the pond" of incense. The size of the pond from which the topic and practice of incense spans is not a small pond, but rather, is worldwide. It is my hope, that in dipping into this pond, your senses will be reignited. The sense of smell is only one potential key to the opening of our awareness to the grandeur of the world. Others offered by *The Incense Bible* include a glimpse at the amazing world of plants and their relationships to human beings, the development of spirituality, and an appreciation of the cultures that make up the world.

It is important to note, as we begin our journey into the world of incense, that this book is intended to focus on authentic natural incense, not the synthetic fragrance-dipped incense to which most of us are accustomed. Integral in this discussion of the relevance of incense to our lives is the importance of the sense of smell, which is addressed in Chapter 2. Why has the sense of smell been so abandoned? Perhaps in an age when more and more people are questioning their purpose in life and connection to the divine, it is timely that this sense, sometimes called the most sacred of our senses, is beginning to get some credence. In fact, as I was writing this book, the Nobel Peace Prize in Physiology or Medicine (2004) was awarded to researchers of the sense of smell. Richard Axel, of Columbia University in New York, and Linda Buck, of the Fred Hutchinson Cancer Research Center in Seattle won the prize by describing the genes that give us our sense of smell.

Another important note for the readers of this book is that this book is not intended to favor any particular religion, spirituality, or ritual. Rather, the book includes a glimpse of some of those beliefs and rituals that I was lucky enough to learn something about in my research of this incredibly broad and important topic. We, as human beings, have followed the scent of incense through the ages, and across the globe for many reasons. In many cases it is possible to see how the

The Incense Bible
© 2007 by The Haworth Press, Inc. All rights reserved.
doi:10.1300/5820_a

use of certain types of incense was borrowed from one culture or type of religion and used in another, and in other cases it is clear that the use of incense coevolved on its own independently. The use of incense is an ancient practice, one that reaches further back than the written history of man and woman, with meaning in people's lives still today.

The Incense Bible includes a look at specific types of incense-producing plants (Chapter 4). However, many others were not included. It is my hope that the discussion of the plants included increases the general awareness of authentic incense and the plants that produce it, the efforts made in its sustainable production, and the sustainable income-generation opportunities available among rural and indigenous peoples.

Last, I hope that you, the reader, can take something home from your glimpse into the world of incense. I hope that the incense is able to furl around your senses and awaken them, and leave you feeling appreciative, fulfilled, and connected by this gift that the plants have given us.

Acknowledgments

I would like to thank the many teachers in the world who are teaching us how to take care of the earth and one another. Many thanks to all those who have shared their incense knowledge with me, including Chief Phil Crazybull, Rufino Paxi, Heng Sure, Steve Stuckey, Father Thomas Scirghi, Connie Grauds, Dr. Ira, Krisa Fredrickson, and Reimar Bruening. A special acknowledgement to Krisa Fredrickson, who has generously shared her library with me. A wish of success for Rufino Paxi, from the Amuta tradition (Bolivia), whose life's work is traveling village to village to teach the Old Ways. A special blessing to the life work of Mestres Acordeon, Suelly, and Rã.

Chapter 1

The Most Spiritual Use of Plants

Incense is not for humans; it is food for the gods.

Mohan Rai, Kirati shaman and shamanism mediator
from Müller-Ebeling et al., 2000

With the morning star guiding their way, the caravan plodded along, cutting a winding trail into the blank canvas of sand. Tassels shook and hooves knocked in the otherwise silent desert. The heat of the day was just hours away, and with it came the danger of transporting the valuable cargo along the trade routes. Battles were fought and people died for this most ancient of plant products—incense.

How is it that something with such a long and rich history, that is present in almost every major religion, can go almost completely unnoticed and undiscussed? Explore the far corners of the world, and incense use is sure to be there. From the Catholic priest swinging incense-filled censers down the aisles of a church in Rome, to the billows of incense smoke that cloud and curl around the Buddha icons in a Buddhist temple in Thailand, to cedar and sweetgrass smoke that fills a Native American sweat lodge in South Dakota—we have been using incense to connect to divinity in almost every culture and class of society for as long as we can look back in time (see Photos 1.1, 1.2, and 1.3).

A WORLDWIDE RITUAL

I believe that incense may be the most spiritual way we use plants across cultures. Almost every major world religion and many smaller, tribal spiritualities light plant parts in worship to seek greater connec-

The Incense Bible
© 2007 by The Haworth Press, Inc. All rights reserved.
doi:10.1300/5820_01

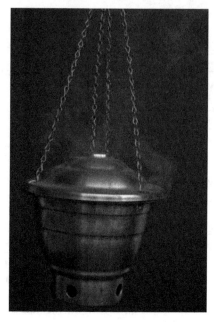

PHOTO 1.1. A censer, also called a thurible, with frankincense and myrrh resin incense smoldering, as used in a Catholic church.

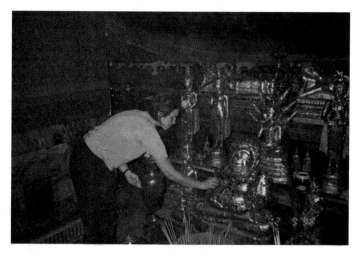

PHOTO 1.2. Author Kerry Hughes at a Buddhist temple in Thailand with incense offering.

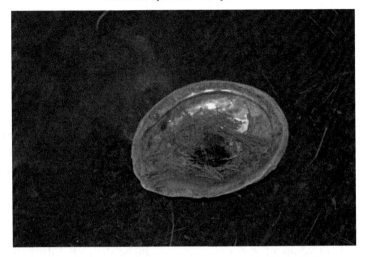

PHOTO 1.3. Flat cedar and sage in an abalone shell.

tion to the divine. Even outside of "religious" use, many people light incense sticks in the home just for the sweet smell and the ability it has to transform space. We may not remember why we started doing it, but unconsciously we know the strength of this ritual.

This book will take you on a tour of the many aspects of incense use, and hope to answer questions about why we do it, where we do it, what greater meanings it assumes, and how can you best use it at home. Incense use is a very broad subject due to its pervasiveness in many cultures, and for this reason this book is not intended to be a comprehensive analysis or account of its use—it is merely multiple dips in the pond.

I expect this book will also run into trouble and question in many of your minds, as spirituality is a deeply personal and controversial topic. This book favors no religion or spiritual practice over another, and the examples that are given are simply those that I have been fortunate enough to find material on, observe, or learn something about. I am no master in this realm, and it is only my deep love for plants and my personal connection with nature and divinity that has driven me to write on these subjects. As an ethnobotanist, I have been fortunate to have had experiences traveling to many areas of the world to learn the ways different cultures and people interact with plants. Although I had never studied incense use formally before writing this book, I always used incense at home and I always collected incenses for my own personal curiosity and use when visiting plant markets in various corners of the globe. I have found these collected incenses to be the greatest reminders of the beautiful lands far away and cultures I have encountered.

I have also felt that incense use is one of the most beautiful and spiritual uses of plants throughout history and still today. Having my deep love of plants, I have often mused how there really couldn't be a more symbolic way to honor the divine as to offer fragrant plants. I have also wondered how others view incense, and have included interviews with various spiritual leaders in this book. Though the reasons for using incense vary considerably throughout different religions and areas of the world, I have found many repeating themes and will discuss them in this book. For me, it seems to be a good way for people to develop a greater connection and respect for nature as they honor divinity through incense, and gain a greater appreciation for what nature has given us.

HONORING THE DIVINITY IN NATURE

With the emerging trends of the lifestyles of health and sustainability, of which 30 percent of the population is said to follow, it seems apparent that many people are walking around this life looking for "connection." They may not be able to articulate what it is they seek, and often this desire is misplaced in overindulgence in materialism, food, alcohol, smoking, or drugs, among other things. As our lives become faster and more surrounded by the urban landscape, it is becoming harder for people to take the time to find out what that desire for connection is all about. Our connection with divinity and nature is not a luxury, and not something that should take a lot of money to cultivate. Our desire for connection is a natural part of who we are as humans, and without it we become unhealthy, diseased, and even perverted. Heng Sure, PhD a Buddhist monk from Berkeley, California, explains that the Buddha's description of the world is related to his experience in meditation, "It [meditation] survived because when other people meditated the way he did, they experienced the same thing—and that is that it [the world] is really ALIVE!" (Sure, personal communication, December 2, 2003).

Our connection with nature is health, and nature supplies us with the vital energy that we need to remain healthy. We all know this innately, and it is very obvious to all of us once we spend a little time in nature. Nature calms and reassures us, and fills us with the vitality of all the life around us. But how can you gain a connection with nature when you live in the city? You don't need to give up your modern luxuries and move out to the country—or even become a hippie! People feel this connection in many ways—from spending time in nature, or through religion and spirituality, to spending time with family or children. These types of activities are part of human nature. This book is not a guide on how to cultivate this connection, but I would like to highlight incense as just one of the aids people use to feel this connection.

The nature of incense—its qualities of being somewhat ethereal, of this world but yet not of this world, here and yet gone, tangible and yet intangible—represents the great mystery of life that we all seek in spirituality. It is a way of gaining an understanding about this mystery and also paying reverence to it. As people burn incense they use their senses and they often ponder the great mysteries of life. Incense is also a way we can invite the divinity that is in all of life and nature into our daily spiritual practice. Even if we live in the city, we can light incense and try to cultivate that connection. The Native American Sioux (hereafter referred to as Lakota)—even those who live in the cities—use incense (called "medicines" or smudges) in their ceremonies, and when they do this they say we are *mitakuye oyasin*—we are all related (see Photo G.1 in the color photo gallery).

This is perhaps the most important understanding for gaining that feeling of connection: to understand that we are all related. Not just the many races of humans on the planet, but also the members of nature—the animals, the plants, the insects—are all here to live life with us, and we are all connected to the divine.

As Heng Sure explains,

> Most of the time (and cognitive science proves this) we have to limit the amount of data that we can process with our six senses. For instance, [if we didn't] how could we drive a car? When we meditate we are tuned in to the senses more. And this makes us aware of how we are in a fabric of existence. So being awake the way that Buddha was awake is a process of not struggling amidst this process, but at the same time not dominating, not

having to have it "my way." The Buddha's prime thing that he awakened to is that the self is just a construct. The "me" in the middle—separate and broken—is just a way of seeing it, and you can practice not seeing it. So when you meditate you awaken to your true self. And this true self is your Buddha-nature. Other religions have other words for this, but it is the concept that you are connected. (Sure, personal communication, December 2, 2003)

If you seek that connection and you aren't sure where to start, perhaps lighting a good quality stick of incense and then sitting down to enjoy it and ponder it is a good start (see Photo G.2 in the color photo gallery). Think about what the plant that it comes from must have looked like, then close your eyes and think about how the scent makes you feel. Think about what paradise means to you and what would it look like. Is it filled with fragrant plants? Then clear your mind and try not to think at all. Do any messages pop into your mind? Imagine you are connected with all of the green trees and beautiful parts of nature you have seen before. Try to feel the love you hold for all of this beauty, and take it with you throughout your day.

UNIFICATION OF MIND, BODY, AND SPIRIT

Beyond our sense of connection that we need to be healthy, incense can also help us to garner awareness and align ourselves in mind, body, and spirit. As incense signifies elements of the spirit realm, it is often used as a medicine and for healing in traditional healing systems throughout the world. If you have ever been to an acupuncturist that has used moxa on you, then you have experienced the use of incense in medicine (see Photo 1.4). As the mind is inseparable and a very useful part of healing the body, so is spirit considered to have an inseparable role in the healing of our physical and mental illnesses in many cultures.

Many people who live the busy Western lifestyle are unaware of this connection, and go about their lives feeling as if they are a "head" with a body that is attached but separated from the daily functions of the mind. With yoga's emergence as a popular new "workout trend" in the United States, many people are discovering for the first time that their minds and bodies *are* connected. The thoughts and emo-

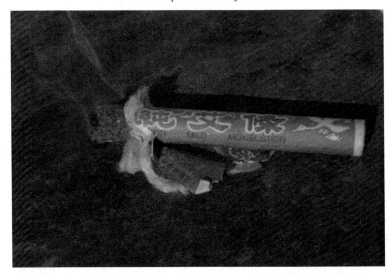

PHOTO 1.4. A moxa stick as used for moxibustion within traditional Chinese medicine.

tions that run around in our heads daily affect our health and the way we feel. By gaining awareness first, and then access to this connection, we may improve our overall health and help prevent several of the typical Western diseases, such as high blood pressure. Many people use meditation or yoga to cultivate the connection between mind and body, but incense can play a role in this as well.

Just as the mind-body connection is important to health, so is our connection with spirit, according to many traditional healing systems. Many more primitive and ancient healing systems throughout the world have a type of doctor that is a doctor-priest. They may be called witch doctors, shaman, or *curanderas,* but in any case they are healers that appeal to the spirit dimension in the healing of disease. To such individuals, illness is believed to have a spiritual component, and taking medicine alone is usually not the only prescribed course of treatment. In the various rituals and methods that these healer-priests use, incense is an important medicine. It often is used for chasing away bad energies or spirits, attracting good ones, and protecting the patient and healer in the course of healing. The use of incense in healing is a deep topic, but it is a key topic to mention when understanding the importance of incense to the many aspects of our selves.

WHAT IS INCENSE?

We have all seen incense sticks, and many of us have ideas of what incense use is or isn't depending on our exposure to its popular use or various spiritual rituals. Many people who have been to a Roman Catholic church may have witnessed the swinging of censers down the aisle, filling the church with sweet-smelling resins. Others in the Western world may have a stigma connecting incense sticks and illegal drug use. This may be because "head shops" carry synthetically fragranced incense sticks that marijuana smokers and psychedelic aficionados like to use to cover up the smell of pot. Still others may have tried the incense sticks in the home for scenting the air, and found them to be too smoky, irritating to the eyes and nose, and nothing like the fragrant descriptions on the package, and thus decided never to light one again. However, incense *sticks* are not the same as pure, clean, raw incense. Raw incense is just that—raw plant parts that are usually dried and ready for use for burning to release fragrant smoke. In addition, although good quality natural incense is available in stick or cone form, most of the incense we buy on the shelf is of very poor quality and made with synthetic fragrances. Vast differences exist between incense sticks that are made from natural oils and resins and ones that are made from synthetic oils and mixtures, as the vast majority are these days.

Incense is defined as a material that is burned to produce an odor, usually fragrant, and is also referred to as the perfume or fumigation itself that is produced from the burning of plant or other materials (Bedini, 1994).

Incense comes in different forms. In its most simple unprocessed form, it is parts of plants that are dried and somehow combusted to produce a fragrant smoke. These plant parts may be pieces of bark, stem, root, leaves, or even resins (plant sap) (see Photos G.3 and G.4 in the color photo gallery, and Photos 1.5 and 1.6). Some of these raw forms of incense can be combusted easily with a match, such as a leaf of dried sage. Others, such as frankincense resin, have to be placed on charcoal, a hot stone, or processed with a saltpeter mixture to create a smoldering effect that causes the resin to release its scent.

This book will focus on the raw incense types and the various uses and reasons we use incense. As an almost unlimited number of blends of incense exists, to cover these would be a lengthy topic and not

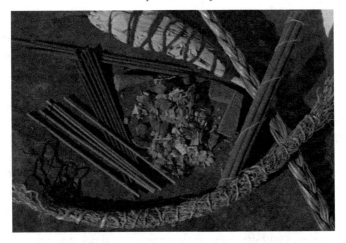

PHOTO 1.5. Various natural incense forms, as seen on the book cover. Natural incense sticks and cones are available, but they are not common.

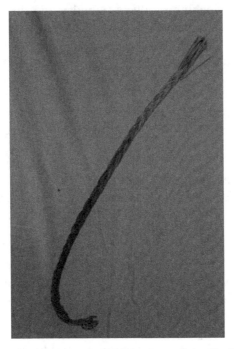

PHOTO 1.6. A grasslike incense (sweetgrass) that is braided and then burned over charcoal or hot rocks, or is lit at the end.

suited for the purpose of this book. The purpose of this book, rather, is to get us all thinking about incense use and how it fits into spiritual- ity, and to reintroduce us to pure raw or natural incense—the incense that is not adulterated or made of synthetic fragrance.

The common forms of processed incense that we are familiar with are incense sticks and cones. If they were the real, natural product they would contain some mixture of raw incense (resins, stems, leaves, bark, etc.), sometimes with added pure essential oils. This then would be mixed together with a base wood material containing saltpeter (potassium nitrate) (not as natural), or a natural alternative for saltpeter, such as a careful mixture of resins and wood, and then dipped onto sticks (usually bamboo splints) or formed into cones.

The more common incense product on the market these days, how- ever, contains synthetic oils, fragrances, and dyes that are really not the same as the pure natural products. Synthetic fragrances have taken over our surroundings and are added to myriad everyday prod- ucts, including cleaning products (laundry and dishwashing deter- gents, wood polish, bleach), cosmetic and body care products (de- odorants, nail polish remover, talcum powder, lotions, shampoo, perfume), and air fresheners (car fresheners, plug-in home fragrance, sprays, potpourris). We are so barraged by the scent of synthetic product fragrance that common scents (either synthetic or natural) sometimes trigger the thought of a commercial product. For example, many people who smell lemon rinds may think of wood polish imme- diately (Aftel, 2001). This has caused many of us displeasure from our sense of smell, and therefore many of us have unconsciously trained ourselves to avoid the simple pleasures of scent. The good news is that we can learn how to trust this sense again, and start at one of the most primitive types of fragrance. Incense use can teach us to be more sensual and spiritual people, and connect us to the divine or the divinity of nature—which is something we all need to stay healthy. The use of incense is a beautiful ritual that is used throughout cultures of the world, and is something that can bring awareness, a feeling of wellness, and a connectedness to anyone who uses it.

The effects of scents such as incense on our sense of smell is inte- gral to understanding our connection with incense; therefore, we will later discuss the relation of our sense of smell to our experiences, di- vinity, and history.

A QUICK TOUR OF INCENSE HISTORY

It is not known when or why the first plants were used as incense, but in ancient cultures of the East incense use has a long association with death. It is theorized that the use of fragrant woods in funeral pyres, which were used to cover the offensive smells of cremation, may have been one of the earliest examples of incense use. In later years, the resins and gums of fragrant woods, such as frankincense and myrrh, were also used in temples, at least in part to cover the stench of burning human and animal offerings. It is thought that later incense gained religious significance and then was used for gaining spiritual enlightenment (Bedini, 1994).

The normal story of the history of incense is that it originated in Egyptian or Babylonian times. Arabia, home to frankincense and myrrh, became the main supply route to the rest of the world. India has long been thought of as the mecca of the fragrant incenses, as Hindu, Muslim, and Buddhist spiritual practices were spread to other areas carrying Indian incense blends. It is also normally told that incense came to China through the spread of Buddhism from India, yet evidence exists of incense use in China before this time (Bedini, 1994; Atchley, 1909).

In this normal history of incense, it is also often said to have originated from the Garden of Eden—a true paradise. The Garden of Eden is said to have existed in Mesopotamia, the "Land of Two Rivers." This ancient land of Asia Minor was situated between the Tigris and Euphrates rivers, and was described as possessing natural enchanted beauty. Since the inhabitants of ancient Mesopotamia were at the convergence of four major trade routes, and the population of the area practiced incense burning daily, the area developed a highly refined incense-burning culture. Later, Abraham brought this knowledge of incense use to the Holy Land, and the Mesopotamian incense traditions permeated Christianity (Fischer-Rizzi, 1996).

I believe that an untold story exists that would reveal the true origin of incense. Incense use, although not always called "incense," has been present in most human cultures from very far back in time, farther back than recorded history can trace. The usual history of incense assumes all incense to be those kinds commonly found on the market. However, incense materials have been found to have been in use in many other cultures, possibly from farther back in history. Incense even now is still found in almost all corners of the globe, and it is not the incense that comes from India, but usually a locally grown plant that is burnt and offered in divine worship and healing. Chapter 3 will highlight some of the areas where incense has been used in religions and spirituality throughout the world.

The history of our sense of smell is also important to understanding the history of incense, as smell is not just something that affects us biologically and psychologically—it is something that is expressed and experienced culturally (Classen et al., 1994). Can one of our five senses help us gain that connection we seek, and help us to understand the great mysteries of life and divinity around us? Chapter 2 examines these aspects of the sense of smell and explores why it has been called the "sacred sense."

IS INCENSE SAFE?

"Even if used daily, incense burning never does harm." In the very ancient yet sophisticated Japanese incense tradition, called *Koh-do,* there are ten virtues of incense burning (summarized by a Zen priest in the sixteenth century), one of which refers to its safety. Beyond being safe, the virtues described the burning of incense as healthful for our spirit and person in several different ways (Fischer-Rizzi, 1996). See Chapter 5 for more information.

According to a report performed by the EPA to examine the potential of candles and incense as sources of indoor air pollution, burning incense and candles can be a source of particulate matter. In addition, in their review of the literature, the EPA linked incense smoke exposure of certain brands of incense to several illnesses. Some incenses are even thought to cause skin irritation, and reportedly have mutagenic and asthma-aggravating effects (Knight et al., 2001).

According to Rufino Paxi (Paxi, personal communication, May 22, 2004), a traditional healer and medicine man of the Ayamara, a culture of the Bolivian Andes, not all the incenses are meant for indoors, and some can even be harmful if used this way. He says people often don't understand this, and buy a number of different incenses that are synthetic or contain natural compounds that are dangerous. Of the incenses available in the high Bolivian marketplace, he says copal is the best, and is good for you. He says the copal he uses is so safe that it may sometimes be used internally (prepared as a traditional medicine) to treat certain illnesses (see Photo G.5 in the color photo gallery).

Many of the allergic reactions or irritations that are suffered from incense, however, come from burning incense with artificial oils. For example, in an article in the peer-reviewed journal *Contact Dermatitis,* a Japanese man in his sixties had come to a clinic with an itchy skin irritation on his body. It was known that he had practiced the Japanese incense ceremony *(Koh-do)* for fifteen years with no problems, however when they did patch testing it was found that perfume added to the incense was the cause of the dermatitis. The physicians in the clinic hypothesized that the perfume in the incense must have become airborne when it was burnt, and then caused the dermatitis when the volatilized particles came in contact with his skin (Hayakawa et al., 1987).

Beyond the various linkages of incense, particularly synthetics, to illness, numerous reports are building about the healing and therapeutic qualities of incense. Perhaps the best way to view this conflicting information is to consider incense as something that is best used in its natural form, and then to also use it in a responsible way. As with other herbal medicines, incense may have the potential for abuse and overindulgence, which may result in certain side effects. In addition, if you are a person with sensitive skin or asthma, it may be wise to limit your incense use, or start by using only pure kinds of incense in small quantities.

Heng Sure explains that incense is the earth element going through the air. According to Sure,

> There is more to incense than the smoke. This is an esoteric and funny thing, but sometimes I am aware of the incense right before I light it. There is an essence or some pervasiveness that happens just as or before it lights, and if you wait for the smoke, that is more crude. There is a transformation where fire releases something in the incense that is connected already as it transforms. The Buddhists would say that as soon as you move to offer the incense, it is already connected and the Buddhas are not waiting for the smoke to curl up, they are waiting for the intent. So the incense becomes a vehicle. (Sure, personal communication, December 2, 2003)

This is a good explanation of why you don't need much incense to enjoy its benefits if you are sensitive to the smoke.

This book focuses on the pure, true, raw forms of incense. It is my hope that people will be able to distinguish between the artificial types of incense on the market and the many benefits and long tradition of use of the pure incense materials. Chapter 2 will discuss the natural versus synthetic scents, and some of the differences in their effects. This book does not promote or condone the use of artificial scents either as incense or as perfume.

TYPES OF RAW INCENSE

What kinds of incense are the pure, true incenses on which this book is focused? Chapter 4 gives an introduction to several kinds of incense from around the world, including agarwood, balsam of Peru/ Tolu, benzoin, camphor, cedar, copal, dragon's blood, eucalyptus, frankincense, mugwort, myrrh, sandalwood, sweet grass, vetiver, and white sage (see Photos G.27-G.28 in photo gallery). These specific incenses were chosen so they may serve as examples of the true worldwide phenomena of incense use. Incense use has apparently developed repeatedly in cultures that could have had no contact. In this way, it shows the universal spiritual quality of incense use. These incense plants produce incense materials, which include resins, leaves, bark, stems, etc., that are used as incense or in the manufacture of incense.

The incense that most of us are familiar with are the incense sticks that are found in numerous specialty shops that carry items for the home, such as scented candles. However, incense is available in a number of forms, including bundles, sticks, cones, rods, coils, small blocks, wands, braids, ropes, and powders. You may buy one of these manufactured forms of incense, choose to use a more raw material form of incense (such as burning resin straight on charcoal), or you may want to learn to make your own.

HOW CAN I USE INCENSE?

Incense use comes from numerous areas in the world, and perhaps the best way to experiment with incense is to find incense that is local to your area of the world. Find incense to buy that is pure and from a reliable manufacturer, or use incense that is particular to your spiritual or religious beliefs. Incense use has many purposes. You must find a purpose for yourself. Reasons for using incense include for the simple aroma, for the mind-body connection, to perfume the hair and clothes, for meditation, for prayer and divine worship, finding vision and dreams, for a feeling of connectedness, as a sacrifice, for cleansing/purification, for healings, for creative inspiration, to improve the mood or learning and problem solving, for lovemaking, for inducing sleep, for marking seasons and rites, and finally in death, in remembrance, and to help the soul make a break from the body.

While teaching me about the qualities of cedar incense (or smudge) and its ability to help us find vision, Chief Phil Crazybull, Native American medicine man and Chief of the Lakota, explained to me the importance of living not only in your vision but in your dream:

> To live in vision, we say that the creator gave us eyes, and with these eyes every day is a living vision. If we were born in darkness and we had to dream everything, then we would have to live by that. But the Creator gave us eyes to see to show us that "this is your living vision—this is your dream, this is what I have given you; this is your living vision." That is why you can see another person, that is why you can see things, that is why you can create things, that is why you are part of human life—and every day is a living vision. And at nighttime when you dream of how you are going to conduct your life, or you want to help somebody in your life, it is related to the dreams of what you want to do with your life [your calling]. (Chief Crazybull, personal communication, February 2004)

The last chapter of this book is dedicated to helping you find your particular connection to incense and the ritual or use that is right for you. Perhaps you will read this book and gain an understanding and appreciation for the finer incenses, and burn them in your home just for a pleasant smell and the atmosphere it creates. Or maybe you will find deeper meaning in it, as many religions and types of spirituality around the world have. Whatever use you choose, I hope it will help to connect you to your dreams and to the earth in a special way.

Chapter 2

The Sacred Sense

A day without fragrance is a day lost.

Ancient Egyptian saying

Search your mind and memory for what you remember to be your favorite smell (see Photo 2.1). Could it be roses? Maybe the smell of newly fallen snow in the wintertime? The aroma of your favorite dish cooking on the stove? The scent of your lover? Now, try to describe that smell in words.

Did you say that roses smell sweet? Or they smell like perfume? Does the snow smell clean, crisp, or cold? Does your favorite dish smell savory or spicy? How about your lover, does he or she smell like their favorite perfume/cologne, or just like themselves? It's not so easy to describe, and what do these terms have anything to do with the sense of smell itself?

Did you notice how your descriptive terms were each like something else, or described as a taste, or a feeling ("crisp, cold")? The sense of smell has an important characteristic when compared to our other senses: we have no language to describe it. We are able to describe the way we see things (by color, shape, texture, etc.), feel things (by texture, temperature, etc.), taste things (sweet, spicy, hot, cold, bitter, pungent, sour, etc.), and hear things (loud, soft, shrill, whisper, etc.). But the only way to describe the things we smell is by naming other objects that we have smelled before, or using the descriptions of our other four senses (for example, "it smells sweet"). Because we have no way of describing it—a common characteristic to our relationship with other sacred objects—there is a divinity to the sense of smell. That is why it is often called our *sacred sense* (Ackerman, 1990; Classen et al., 1994).

The Incense Bible
© 2007 by The Haworth Press, Inc. All rights reserved.
doi:10.1300/5820_02

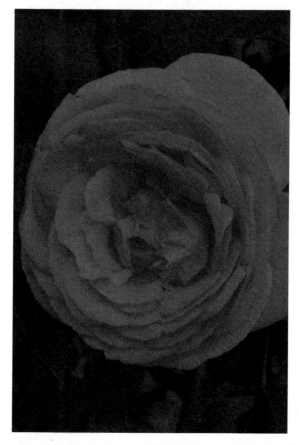

PHOTO 2.1. An old-fashioned rose. Old-fashioned varieties of flowers and plants were selected and favored for their abundant fragrance, whereas those today are selected for other features, such as shelf life and what looks good in a nursery container.

What about the emotions that each of these scents evoke? Close your eyes and imagine being in an embrace with your lover. As you nuzzle your face in the nape of his or her neck, are you aware of your feelings as you inhale the scent? Have you ever kept an article of your lover's clothing at your side when he or she is away on a trip? Do you take a whiff of his or her shirt and instantly feel as if you are in that embrace, right there at that very moment?

The sense of smell has the magical ability of transporting us to memories of the past that no other sense does as completely. It is as if that old blanket from your grandma can transport you instantaneously into her house, visiting as a child, and you can suddenly remember everything in vivid detail—the texture of the couch, her face as she is sitting across from you knitting, how it feels to be that age again.

Our memories betray us as we get older. They slowly erode, and try as we might it is difficult to recall the happy moments, exciting dreams, and important people in our lives. Scent is our magical time machine, a transport vehicle that goes straight to the oldest part of our evolved brains, and is able to somehow, and instantly, make us not only remember but to see, feel, taste, and maybe even hear those memories. Perhaps it may also transport us to more distant times, other lives or an ancient feeling or memory of what it means to be human. These qualities are what give the sense of smell a divinity, or sacredness.

Scents and the sense of smell have been present with us throughout time and have pervaded themselves into how we perceive time; how we express our spirituality and religious traditions; how we classify or perceive one another, both between genders and between classes; how we seduce our lovers; how we manipulate commercial products' seductiveness; and how we reach higher levels of consciousness and healing. The history of our sense of smell also contains shocking revelations about how we have denigrated this natural sense to become that of the primitive and uncivilized, giving rise to the popularity of synthetics.

SCENT THROUGH TIME

Smell is not something that affects us only biologically and psychologically—it is something that is expressed and experienced culturally. Smells have social and historical values that often change through time with a culture, and what is described as fragrant or smelling good may be perceived quite the opposite by another culture. Studying what it is to smell has even been described as studying what is the very essence of human culture. Smells are often permeated with cultural codes and conduct, and they are internalized by the people of that culture in very personal ways. They are not usually thought of consciously, but reacted to physically. In other words, we may not even be able to describe our beliefs about certain odors, but those beliefs are held so deeply in us that they become embodied by us, and we may react to them in a very physical way (Classen et al., 1994).

In shocking words George Orwell characterizes what "the real secret" is in the class differences between upper and lower classes in the modern West—it is that "the lower classes smell." What more personal way of experiencing class differences is there than through the sense of smell? In this sense, the division the upper class feels toward the lower class becomes actually physical, repulsive, and this automatic biological repulsion is not something that can be changed easily. At the same time, this statement is characteristic of the modern Western cultural perspective of scent. The sense of smell has been devalued, and has become thought of as a barbaric and undesirable sense. In the late nineteenth century, scents went through what was termed an "olfactory revolution." Scents—that once held an important position in science and medicine—were devalued in these areas and moved exclusively to the realms of sentiment and sensuality, and were left to the "frivolousness of women" (Classen et al., 1994).

To gain an understanding of how we got to this point—the absence of fragrance or preferential use of synthetic fragrances being culturally valued over natural scents—it is important to understand the natural history of scents through the cultures that led up to the modern Western times.

SCENTS IN ANCIENT AND CLASSICAL TIMES

Roman and Greek gods were thought to not only favor certain sweet odors, but also to emit them. Zeus was described as living atop a fragrant cloud, and when Hera went to seduce him she bathed her entire body in an ambrosial oil. None of the Greek or Roman gods were more connected to scent than the goddess of love, Aphrodite (or Venus). She was said to live in a fragrant temple, with attendants that anointed visitors in ambrosia (Classen et al., 1994).

Scented items then were used as not only an offering to the gods, but also were used to signal their presence. There was no division between scents that were secular and those that were sacred, and the gods were assumed to be fond of all the same smells that mortals liked. However, the gods were also thought to be quite fond of the odor of burnt animal offerings. Back then animals of all sorts were sacrificed and burnt in a ceremonial offering to the gods. This ceremony, however, was always accompanied by incense, perhaps to mask the unpleasantness of the stench (Classen et al., 1994).

Incense was the standard offering to the gods of those times, and it often constituted the whole offering, with no other sacrifices. In the sixth century BC the Pythagorean cult believed that animals had a soul and also the right to live as much as we did. They believed that animal sacrifice was therefore wrong, and promoted incense as an alternative offering. Other offerings included flowers and perfumes. Among the common rituals was the perfuming of statues of sacred icons, as well as decorating them with garlands of flowers. As people also enjoyed those scents, and felt gods favored them when they were scented, they used perfume and flower garlands for their bodies as well (Classen et al., 1994).

In these times, the place where the gods resided, Mount Olympus, was believed to be a place of fragrance, in contrast to the earth where the mortals lived, which was marked by the scent of decay and corruption. This general belief was carried on through the Middle Ages in the beliefs of Christianity, with all that is sinful and worldly being associated with foul odor. This association is repeated through many cultures, including in Islamic belief (Classen et al., 1994).

CHRISTIANITY AND THE ODOR OF SANCTITY

In a similar manner to the odors that were associated with the gods of classical times, in Christianity evolved the belief of a holy scent that signaled the presence of the Holy Spirit. The presence of this mystical fragrance of the Holy Spirit could also be found in people who were thought to be favored by God, or it could also be thought of as a sign of their personal holiness. Indeed, priests of the early Christian tradition were all thought to possess this fragrance—a thought which may have had some relation to the rose garlands worn by the priests, and the burning of incense that was so common in that time (Classen et al., 1994).

Certain priests and saints were well noted to emit the "odor of sanctity," and upon death they would emit it even stronger. It was as if these holy people were above the decay of mortality, and as their spirit left their bodies the sweet scent only exhibited their incontrovertible holiness. A couple examples of this are the fifth century monk Simeon Stylites, later designated a Saint, who emitted a sweet fragrance as he performed the ascetic act of living on top of a pillar away from earthly temptations, and as he got ill and died, the scent grew only stronger and stronger. The seventeenth century Venerable Benedicta of Notre-Dame-du-Laus was also known for her divine scent. This sweet scent was known to be emitted not only from her and her clothing, but all that she touched was as if it had been perfumed (Classen et al., 1994).

One literal explanation of these beliefs was the statement from St. Paul that "we are the aroma of Christ to God among those who are being saved and those who are perishing" (2 Corinthians 2:15; New International Version). It is also true that early Christianity included the use of much incense, rose garlands, and the burying of corpses (mostly of the wealthy) with herbs and spices. However, in cases when the odor of sanctity was emitted upon a death, reports stated that no herbs or spices were used in the burial in order to dismiss any suspicion of this. St. Isidore was said to show no signs of decay and to emit a strong sweet odor of sanctity when his body was exhumed forty years after his death, and then once more 150 years after his death the fragrance was emitted when the corpse was moved to another tomb (Classen et al., 1994).

The odor of sanctity showed the ideal concept of the mark of holiness of that time, whereas moral corruption and things associated with the devil were thought to reek of the stench of the devil. The devil himself was thought to emit a strong stench of sulfur, and sins and sinners were thought to embody malodors of almost any kind (Classen et al., 1994).

THE "OLFACTORY REVOLUTION"

In the end of the nineteenth century, as previously mentioned, an "olfactory revolution" took place that completely changed our relationship with the sense of smell. At that time the cities of Europe had become so stench-ridden that it is a wonder why anyone would want to live in the city. The populations of the cities grew, and both garbage and sewer disposal were unplanned and out-of-control problems. To add to this, the cholera and typhus epidemics of the nineteenth centuries spawned fear as many people suspected odors to be a cause of spreading the diseases. Therefore, sanitary reform that had been so badly needed began to finally take hold, mostly due to this fear (Classen et al., 1994).

To illustrate what the European cities might have been like, it is possible to draw from the works of writers who were advocates of a reform to cleanliness, who then took it upon themselves to document the horror of the stench and uncleanliness of the cities. The horrors of the Fleet River in London were captured in a poem called "On the Famous Voyage" by poet Ben Jonson. It is a story about two companions taking a boat voyage down the river and describing their encounters along the way, from animal carcasses to human waste (Classen et al., 1994).

Sewage and waste disposal mostly occurred on the streets of the city, which was then washed into the nearby rivers. Everything one would use in the household and want to dispose of was normally just thrown onto the street, from animal carcasses and entrails to organic matter from fruits and vegetables. To make it worse, the "sewers" were usually the side alleys next to houses, or if a house was situated near a river this was used. Many houses of that time had a platform with a hole that was located over the street alley or the river, and this served as the toilet. As the streets in the cities were made of dirt, one can imagine the foul muck that was created as the dirt mingled with garbage and sewage (Classen et al., 1994).

Added to the direct refuse of people, the cities also harbored slaughterhouses in which herds of animals were kept in tight confines, and their manure and waste left to pile up in the yards. In addition, dairies in the cities kept cows on a permanent basis. As herds were led through the cities, cows that fell dead after drinking muck from the gutters were left in the streets to rot and be run over by wagon traffic, as were any dogs or cats that were stray in the city.

The industrial revolution of the late eighteenth century added industrial waste to this stench. Factories sprang up throughout the European cities and strew black fumes from burning coal. The cities became enveloped by this black soot, and it became so strong that it even covered many of the other odors of the city (Classen et al., 1994).

Smoke then was already tolerated in the home, as there was a widespread belief that it made both the home and the inhabitants healthy.

Most houses had a central fire and a simple hole in the roof in order to ventilate the smoke. Therefore, houses were smoky, and they also contained a mixture of both rank and sweet odors. The floors back then were a clay that might be covered continuously by fresh marsh rushes. As the new layer of rushes were added to the top, the bottom was left to degrade along with all that had fallen on it. The spittle, beer dregs, vomit, and urine from dogs or other animals kept in the house in this degrading layer lent a certain stench to any house, that then was covered up by the strewing of sweet herbs and flowers on the floor, or by the use of other perfumes, the burning of aromatic woods, or of herbal bouquets, such as nosegays (bouquets of herbs and flowers that people carried with them and held in front of noses when the stench became strong) (Classen et al., 1994).

The castles of the Middle Ages and the Renaissance that we like to dream about romantically were not made for pleasure, but for keeping the inhabitants safe. Therefore, among the common walls of the castle would be cramped stalls of farm animals, and buildings filled with pitch and sulfur, mixing together in an olfactory stench. In addition, most people in the countryside lived with their farm animals under the same roof (Classen et al., 1994).

When the plagues swept Europe through the fourteenth to seventeenth centuries, new plagues would break out every few years, and this became part of life. Of course, we now know it was the fleas from rats that were the carriers of the plague, but at that time there were many guesses about what might be causing it. Some people believed it to be associated with dogs, since it was during the astrological phenomenon of the dog days of summer that the plague was most active. This was when the strength of the rays of the sun and Sirius, the dog star, were the strongest. As dogs were believed to be causing the plague, some towns had mass slaughterings of dogs in order to lessen it (Classen et al., 1994).

However, by far the most common belief of what was causing the plagues was putrefaction. The belief that odors could carry disease was rationalized in different ways, but it was strengthened by the fact that people with the plague emitted a strong odor. Therefore, cities had municipal burning of aromatic woods to keep the air purified. In homes it was a common protection measure to strew herbs, burn incense and other aromatic herbs and woods, and to use almost any other strong-smelling substances, such as vinegar and gunpowder—

anything to drive away the putrid smell of plague. Likewise, in order to visit a person sick with the plague, a series of perfuming rituals or the carrying of other aromatic spices on the body or in the mouth was recommended (Classen et al., 1994).

To both treat the plague and to prevent it, aromatic substances were most relied upon. This was because the nose was considered, by the medical theory of that time, to give a direct path to the brain and therefore the spirit. As scent was thought to have a similar nature to the spirit, or the life force, scented medications were thought to be the most effective at treating the plague (Classen et al., 1994).

At the start of the "olfactory revolution," scientists of that time observed that animals would writhe and die when kept in a sealed container. Thus it was observed that fresh air was necessary to all life. As the poor lived in cramped conditions, with little fresh air circulation, it was thought that their own exhalations were lethal. This contributed to a growing division between classes based on scents (Classen et al., 1994).

Trying to fix the sanitary problems of the city—now that the problem was agreed upon—was a large task. To make matters more difficult, many poor people relied on the garbage on the street for their income, in such professions as street sweepers, manure sellers, and people who went door-to-door gathering sewage pots. In 1832 there was even a riot over the issue of sanitary reform by poor people in Paris. It took a long time for reform to take hold because, just as today, a clean environment—clean streets—were regarded a luxury, and jobs for the people were regarded a necessity that took precedence. It took the rising deaths from cholera for government to finally put reform measures in place, and then begin house inspections, installation of flush toilets, and the building of sewage systems (Classen et al., 1994).

The discovery in the late nineteenth century that it was germs and not smells that spread disease gave further importance and priority in continuing with the mass building of sewage system projects. As the cities became less soaked by the odor of sewage, the other odors of the city, notably the industrial odors, became more prominent to its inhabitants. Pressure by the urban populations then started industrial waste reforms (Classen et al., 1994).

Along with a mass change in civic cleanliness came a mass change in personal cleanliness. Previously thought to be harmful for the health, bathing became thought of as good for the health, especially after scientists discovered that animals would suffocate and die when their bodies were covered by tar. Since the upper and middle classes were the first to begin bathing, the odors of the working classes became more noticeable. The poor working class not only did not bathe, but their houses were also designed differently. At this point it had become common for houses in the upper and middle classes to separate areas of their households (i.e., separate bedrooms, bathrooms, kitchens, and dining rooms). Therefore, the working classes began to be looked down upon as smelling, and consisting of an "olfactory promiscuity that equated a moral promiscuity" (Classen et al., 1994, p. 82).

As personal cleanliness became more popular, the use of perfumes declined significantly. This was due to a number of factors, including the fact that they were just not needed in as high a volume to mask other unpleasant scents. Perfumes were thought of by some religious people as unclean as any scent, as odors were equated with being morally unclean. Perfumes also began to be thought of as bad for the health, as the merits of washing with waters to free the skin of toxins became more popular. In this way perfumes were thought of as something that might actually clog the pores, and keep the body from detoxifying naturally. As medicine now saw no merit for the use of scented medicaments, they were taken out of the pharmacy and relegated to cosmetic use only (Classen et al., 1994).

Around this time there was also a trend in clothing fashions, as well as perfumes, toward more simplicity. It was no longer seen as desirable to display the frivolous excess of the upper classes. In France, the French Revolution brought a revolt against anything that was seen as aristocratic excess. By the end of the eighteenth century, men stopped wearing perfumes altogether, and women switched to more lighter floral scents. Before this time, perfume was always enjoyed and worn by both sexes, and there was not the division of what was appropriate for men versus women as there later became—a division that has stood through the present time (Classen et al., 1994).

Due to these changes, and the olfactory revolution, the perfume industry capitalized on these trends and began creating scents exclusively for women, and other scents for products that were just for men (aftershave and cologne). In addition, because perfumes were deemed frivolous, serving no purpose in medicine, they became of the realm of women, who were also thought to be frivolous creatures. This was the beginning of our devaluing of scents, and lays the ground for why we use synthetics and why incense has never become a popular topic despite its pervasiveness (Classen et al., 1994).

THE ESSENCE OF CULTURAL, CLASS, AND GENDER DIFFERENCES

In order to further understand why incense has never become a topic worth serious discussion in the West, it is important to understand the deep beliefs of scent in expressing gender and power differences. The American male today is associated with the ideal of having no scent, and women in general are associated with the ideal of having a light flowery scent. Beyond the sexist difference in the culturally bound idea of what is acceptable between men and women, it is clear that the ideal for society and public places in general is the absence of scent. How did this come to be that lack of scent could hold such a strong value, especially among American males?

Classen et al. (1994) explain that the nature of power today is that it is centralized and taken away from the individual. Since power used to be personal it was also associated with the scents and beliefs of those people who had the power. Today, since power is centralized, it has become impersonal and abstract, and therefore without a scent. In the peripheries are women, foreigners, minorities, and the working class, and Classen et al. (1994) explain "that the peripheries smell"— or at least they are perceived that way.

In the case of the genders, there is no clearer example of what is expected culturally than in the case between American men and women. As Classen et al. (1994) explain, the culturally acceptable behavior for American men is to be a "true man"—free from any of the pomp and circumstance of the frivolities of women or men from other cultures. American men see themselves on the whole as being authentic, rugged, and dyed-in-the-wool. Americans as a whole spend more money on perfumes and cosmetics than on education. So, how is it that American men, who dislike scent so much, are attracted to the most perfumed women in the world?

The answer is in the culturally ingrained belief that men are the *choosers* and women are the *chosen*. Women are either believed to be flowery smelling, or putrid and foul smelling by nature. As Classen et al. (1994) explain, whores and prostitutes are characterized as being putrid smelling. In fact, the Latin word for putrid served as the base for the Spanish word for whore, *puta,* and the similar meaning French word, *putain.* The use of perfumes by women is also connected to our idea of the witchlike nature of women, as it is seen to be one of women's lures in order to cast spells over men. However, this idea of women being seductresses, wearing perfume and high heels in order to attract men, has also led to the belief that women are frivolous creatures (Classen et al., 1994).

Other groups that lie in the "periphery" are also thought of as smelling, and this is sometimes used as an expression of disdain. There has never been evidence to prove that races on their own have different discernable smells, and this difference is most probably an imaginary one. However, if any truth exists to differences in certain races or cultures in the odors they emit, it may be due to a few factors. One good explanation may be in the different cuisines consumed by different cultural groups. There has long been an association in the idea that we are what we eat, and that we may take on the scents of the different foods that we eat. Therefore, if a particular cuisine is characterized by a lot of spices, or perhaps a certain kind of meat, it may be possible to effect the odor of the skin and breath. It may also be due to rituals—whether spiritual ones such as using incense or secular ones such as in the nature of bathing—that are specific to cultures (Classen et al., 1994).

What does this have to do with incense? Many people today in the Western culture are sensitive to scents and odor and will outwardly reject to being in their presence. This is a sentiment that was pointed out repeatedly as I visited places of worship and incense use. Are these reactions to scent from the overuse of synthetic scents or from our cultural upbringing? Are we using our sense of smell as a form of prejudice against other cultures and women?

Heng Sure of the Berkeley Buddhist Monastery says that he sees a number of people who when they first come to the monastery object to the scent of incense in the air. He said that one person who was a beginner in meditation even marched into the meditation hall, went to the altar, and without asking put the incense out! As this monastery only uses pure sandalwood, it is hard to imagine that there could have been that unpleasant of a scent in the air.

SEDUCTION AND SCENTS

Scents have always been associated with magic, healing, and sexual power (Classen et al., 1994). Incense—as an early form of scent or perfume—was often used in this way. The use of scents as a lure in sexuality goes back as far as anyone can trace. Scents are sensuous, and it is not only the traditionally thought of musks and florals that are used in the perfume industry that can be used in seduction, but our own bodies produce a complex and individual symphony of scents, by which we most certainly are attracting one another, if not subconsciously.

Cleopatra is often remembered as the ultimate seductress, but some say she was not all that attractive. One of her secrets may lie in the lavish use of scents she employed. She was said to scent her mouth with solid perfume (like a lip gloss) when she kissed a lover, so they would be forced to remember her after their parting. Rumor has it that when she went to receive Mark Antony, she scented the sails of her ship, and they later returned to a room filled with rose petals (Aftel, 2001).

Scents have also been associated with witches, and witchcraft, one of their uses being to ensnare men in love. The use of scents by women as a lure was such a popular conception in Europe that during an act of Parliament in 1770 the use of them by women in order to seduce men became illegal:

> [A]ll women, of whatever age, rank profession, or degree, whether virgins, maids or widows, that shall from and after such Act, impose upon, seduce, and betray into matrimony, any of His subjects, by the scents, paints, cosmetic washes, artificial teeth, false hair, Spanish wool, iron stays, hoops, high-heeled shoes, bolstered hips, shall incur the penalty of the law now in force against witchcraft and like misdemeanors, and that the marriage, upon conviction, shall stand null and void (Classen et al., 1994).

The use of scent in seduction, however, has a very real basis. Pheromones (from the Greek words *pherein,* to transfer, and *horman,* to excite) are substances that are excreted from animals (including us) in order to elicit a physiological and/or behavioral response from others. In humans, they are thought to increase sexual attraction, although some argue that we have lost our ability to detect them with our weakened sense of smell. Perhaps the fact that we are one of the smelliest animals makes this weakened sense of smell an asset instead of a detriment!

Pheromones are detected by most animals by the vomeronasal organ (VNO), and it is the organ by which all cat species gain information about the environment. There is debate as to whether in humans this organ has become vestigial, existing as two small bilateral pits just behind the nostrils. Evidence for them not to be useful in humans is research showing that pheromones can be still detected in people with the VNO removed. But how? Research has found that mice are able to perceive pheromones through their regular olfactory system, indicating that we too may be able to detect pheromones through our sense of smell (Luo et al., 2003; Wysocki et al., 1982).

After we produce pheromones, we make them available to the air on our skin and our sweat. In fact, the hairs in our pubic region and under our armpits serve as tiny antennas in order to hold the scent into the air, and possibly to attract mates to the pubic region. Pheromones are not only made internally, but by the bacteria that live on the skin and hair follicles. Therefore, washing with antibacterial soaps may just cut down on the production of pheromones.

Many kinds of pheromones exist, and each elicit certain physiological responses, many of which we do not know about. In addition, although some "pheromone perfumes" have been available on the market, caution should be taken as to what species those pheromones are produced by, and what physiological effect is elicited by each! It might be wise to figure out whether the pheromone perfume you are wearing is at least one from humans.

One kind of pheromone that has been found in humans is called a copulin, which, as in many species, increases the desire for copulation (you've got to love the humor of scientists). In humans, copulins have been discovered in the vaginal secretions of women around the time of ovulation, which would be an optimal time for the body to want to attract a mate. Men have also been found to secrete pheromones that effect women's mood and responses (Thorne et al., 2002; Chen and Haviland-Jones, 1999). Human pheromone research continues to discover more about our use of pheromones in sexuality. It is becoming clear that in fact we do produce pheromones, and respond to them in terms of sexuality (Cornwell et al., 2004; Silvotti et al.,

2003; Frey, 2003; Thorne et al., 2002; Chen and Haviland-Jones, 1999).

When we are young, we learn about the "birds and the bees." Have you ever mused about how much of the story of the birds and the bees has to do with plants? Plants use scents, as well as many other attractants, such as color and shape, to attract pollinators. To us only a few flowers have distinct scents when compared to the sweet litany of scents that are detectable by insects. Since scent is one of the most important means by which flowers attract pollinators, and thus reproduce, and insects often rely on these flowers for their nectar, pollen, or other rewards, insects have developed an exquisite sense of smell. Have you ever wondered about how those wasps are able to find you just as soon as you start eating outside? A little scent goes a long way for an insect. Sweet-smelling scents are the most general attractants, meaning they will attract a number of different types of insects and birds. Flowers that emit these sweet scents are promiscuous because they can be pollinated by a number of different types of pollinators. Some flowers have scents that are addictive, so that the insects keep coming back for more, while others may open only at night to attract a certain pollinator (such as sphinx moths on evening primroses, or bats on yucca flowers). One plant that is native to California, called the Matilija poppy, has huge poppy flowers (the largest in California) that emit a substance that befuddles bumble bees. As the bumble bee visits the poppy flower, it becomes disoriented due to the substance that is emitted and ends up pollinating the flower through its lingering clumsiness! Other plants produce strange scents, such as the South-African protea, which gives off a strange, yeasty smell in order to attract mice, or the smell of dung or rotting flesh that some carnivorous plants (such as pitcher plants) give off to attract flies and other prey.

The birds and the bees are not the only creatures attracted to sweet floral scents. As women's perfume is normally floral scented, it is clear that it is used to attract human males. Imagine what it might be like if your sense of smell was more acute, and the world was wafting with winds of fragrance and odors. Often we perceive the world to be only as far as our eyes can see, but if our sense of smell was more developed, we could be aware of not only plants, but of people and their activities from far away. Imagine being a cat subjected to catnip! We could be walking along a sidewalk and all of the sudden stop and not be able to resist rolling in our neighbor's shrubs. Like cats, we might roll around in it and smell it all over our bodies as we crush it. We might nibble on it, eat it, rub it against our faces, and then run around uncontrollably, until we returned to the shrub to sleep off our ecstasy. Ah, to be a cat.

Similarly, as scents play this important role in seduction, incense is also used in lovemaking and romance. Chapter 3 describes the use of incense and other scents in the *Kama Sutra,* the Hindu guide to lovemaking. Incense is commonly associated with sensual moments and for creating a mood. Certain incense types, like sandalwood, are described as emitting a sweet and sensuous odor. Perhaps this association is merely related to our ideal of women and floral scents, or perhaps incense is able to awaken that ancient and sensual part of our brains that connects us to our deepest emotions and desires.

SCENTS IN NON-WESTERN CULTURES

Although what is not Western culture is often left out of history—including natural history—traditional and indigenous cultures throughout the world have used scent in their communication and perception of the world from the beginning of time. This is an important realization when studying the worldwide phenomena of incense use and ritual.

Perhaps the most popular example of this role of scent in communication in another culture is "Eskimo kissing," in which people rub their noses together when they meet. There is a theory that the custom of regular kissing (lip to lip) developed in part due to the dual benefit of being able to smell and taste one's partner. Thus, in the Balinese and Eskimo cultures the role of scent becomes even more suspect as an attractive feature by which the custom developed.

Scents play many other roles in various non-Western cultures, from mating and courtship to hunting rituals and beliefs, and from cosmetic and body care to spiritual and religious functions. For example, among the Chewong, aboriginal people from the Malay peninsula, children wear necklaces with ginger attached to them in order to chase away evil spirits; good spirits are attracted and "fed" incense nightly (Classen et al., 1994).

Other cultures often classify and perceive scents in entirely different ways. What might be sweet smelling to once culture may be foul smelling to the members of another culture, and vice versa. For example, the Serer Ndut of Senegal classify scents into five basic categories: urinous, rotten, milky or fishy, acidic or acrid, and fragrant. Only the things belonging to the fragrant category are agreeable scents. They perceive Europeans to be urinous smelling due to infrequent bathing, and to them this is a bad smell. However, it is likely that the Europeans would say the same thing about the Serer Ndut, as they lead a more primitive lifestyle and would be considered part of the "periphery" (Classen et al., 1994).

Differences may also occur in the customs between genders from what we are used to in the Western culture. For example, in Arabia, perfume is not used to mask body odors, but rather to make the body more fragrant and pleasing. Women use perfume and scents more than men, but men do use them as well. Perfumes on women are not for social occasions, as this would seem inappropriate, but rather are more fitted for women to use in the company of their husbands, among other women, or with their families. The use of perfumes by men are limited to generally two fragrances, rose and aloeswood, which may be placed behind the ears, or on the nostrils, beard, or palms of the hands. Both men and women may also scent their clothes with incense, and have special hangers with which to do so (Classen et al., 1994).

Deep differences may also occur in the rituals between the sexes and how this determines one's sexuality. The Hua of the highlands of Papua New Guinea classify gender not only by the individual's genitals, but also be the body's emanations and fluids. Menstruation is thought to hold an evil smell, and the Hua have many rituals and customs around it. During the initiation period of a boy, he takes care not to come into contact with female fluids, as this could impact his masculine identity. In fact, changes in gender are not uncommon among the Hua, as gender identity is so changeable (Classen et al., 1994). This is interesting when compared to the American man's belief that men should not smell flowery like women.

The perception of the importance and role of scent in the natural world may also vary from our culture. For example, among the Wamira of Papua New Guinea, taro roots are believed to dislike certain odors. They believe that when wooden digging sticks are used in their cultivation, the taro is plentiful, and when ordinary metal garden forks are used with rust on them, the plants disappear. Among the Desana of Colombia, hunting is termed "making love to the animals," and hunting involves many specialized rituals that include using an odor with which the hunter makes himself more attractive to the animals. They view hunting like courtship, and the same scents that are used to attract women are also used to attract the animals (Classen et al., 1994).

Although the customs involving scent are often so different around the world, and even the perception of what are good and bad odors, similarities also exist. One of the biggest similarities, which will be developed more fully in Chapter 3, is that incense has been and is used throughout the world in many different cultures for religious and spiritual purposes. How so many cultures in distant areas of the world evolved similar beliefs about the use of incense in spirituality is truly wondrous. Even more wondrous is that many of these incense plant scents are similarly regarded throughout the world, as will be discussed in Chapter 4.

SYNTHETIC VERSUS NATURAL SCENTS

The use of natural scents as incense and perfumes dates back to as far as we can trace in history. Incense has been found to have been heavily used in ancient Egypt, and we know that many other cultures have long oral histories of using natural scents before this. The Egyptians were specifically known to use incense for worship and unguents to rub on the body. They recorded the process of making these scents, and it was clear that scents were highly regarded in their society. After returning from Egypt, Moses was commanded by the Lord to make holy oil using a blend of olive oil and spices. Roman times saw some of the most lavish and abundant uses of scents, perfumes, and incense that have been unsurpassed in history. Indeed, it has been said that during the Age of Discovery, the continents were discovered largely as a result of the quest for aromatics that were used as incense (Aftel, 2001).

An ancient art and science, alchemy has been said to be the root of perfumery. Alchemy has a complex history to trace, and according to some sources its roots go back to ancient China, India, and Egypt. It was considered a calling for the quest of knowing the truth of matter and life. Alchemists believed that the *quinta essentia*—the spark of divinity—could be found in any matter. Once this was understood, then it was believed the alchemist could change the nature of the matter. Alchemists believed that the essential elements of nature were united with the cosmos, and that both the physical and the spiritual were one in unity. They had a belief that "what is above is as that which is below, and what is below is as that which is above." Part of this mystery is that alchemists usually worked alone and shrouded their work in secrecy (Aftel, 2001).

The mysterious alchemists worked with laboratory paraphernalia, and can be credited for refining the process of distillation. Alchemy also gave rise to what is now the modern study of chemistry, and some say that it also gave rise to the modern study of philosophy as it was concerned with harmonizing duality. Early perfumers also kept many of the alchemists' ways, and worked alone and in secrecy (Aftel, 2001).

With the Enlightenment came the "olfactory revolution" that opened the door to a whole new way of approaching scent. In this time the sense of smell became the most undervalued of the senses. Although the sense of smell and odors once played a role in science and scientific theories, with the discovery that it was germs and not odors that carried disease, smell was automatically dismissed by science. At the same time philosophers of the Enlightenment found no way to value scents for aesthetic enjoyment nor as a way of acquiring knowledge. Smell became thought of as a primitive sense because in Darwin's theories of the evolution of man we no longer relied on it, as our noses were now far from the earth and scent trails. In this way the devaluing of the sense of smell became a defining factor for what it meant to be "civilized man" (Classen et al., 1994).

It is interesting that during the writing of this book, two researchers from the U.S. were awarded the Nobel Prize in Physiology or Medicine for discovering the genes that are responsible for our sense of smell. Perhaps the valuation of the sense of smell is evolving again, and incense may become a topic worthy of discussion. Hopefully, our understanding and appreciation of natural scents may then change and we can devalue the prevalence of synthetic scents that are not only present in our incense, but pervasive in the environment around us.

To understand how these synthetics took hold in the world, it is also important to understand the history of perfumery and how synthetic fragrances were developed and valued in the first place. The perfume industry began with the production and fad of wearing scented gloves. In sixteenth-century France, Catherine de Medicis' perfumer, René, both made gloves and had an alchemical laboratory. His retail store and laboratory located in the same building were the first perfume shop in Paris. René was characteristic of an early perfumer who worked with natural scents, and developed an expertise around the complexity and depth of the scents (Aftel, 2001).

As perfumery became more popular, new techniques beyond distillation were developed to capture the scents from the natural raw material (for example, see Table 2.1). One of these was enfleurage, which involved the capture of floral scents that couldn't be distilled into an oil matrix. As the perfume industry grew, new technologies evolved, and the search for new, exciting scents continued, more were added to the repertoire of perfumes. Early blends of perfumes were somewhat unimaginative, as they all strove for the harmony of scents.

TABLE 2.1. Natural scents introduced to perfumery through time (Aftel, 2001).

Ancient scents	Introduced 1500-1540	Introduced 1540-1589	By 1730
Benzoin	Angelica	Basil	Peppermint
Cedarwood	Anis	Melissa	Ginger
Costus root	Cardamom	Thyme	Mustard
Rose	Fennel	Citrus	Cypress
Rosemary	Caraway	Coriander	Bergamot
Sage	Lovage	Dill	Mugwort
Juniperwood	Mace	Oregano	Neroli
Frankincense	Nutmeg	Marjoram	Bitter almo
Cinnamon	Celery	Galbanum	
	Sandalwood	Guaicwood	
	Juniper	Chamomile	
	Black pepper	Spearmint	
		Labdanum	
		Lavender	
		Lemon	
		Mint	
		Carrot seed	
		Feverfew	
		Cumin	
		Myrrh	
		Cloves	
		Opopanax	
		Parsley	
		Orange peel	
		Iris	
		Wormwood	
		Saffron	

However, between 1889 and 1921 in Paris, modern perfumery was born. In these years it became acceptable and new to base fragrance blends not on harmony, but on contrast, and this gave perfumers a whole new way to look at formulation (Aftel, 2001).

The first synthetic scents arrived on the scene toward the end of the nineteenth century. Coumarin was the first to be discovered, which is a natural component in many plants and has the smell of freshly mowed hay. Coumarin was extracted from the tonka bean, and proved to be cheap, stable, predictable, and colorless. The second synthetic to be discovered was vanillin, a component of the vanilla bean (Aftel, 2001).

When the first synthetic scents were discovered, they added only to the creativity of the perfume blends. But then the perfume industry became lured to heavily use synthetics in place of natural scents due to their cheapness, colorlessness, and modernity. Synthetics also eventually allowed for cheap manufacture, as laboratory methods were developed to synthesize the chemicals starting from cheaper petroleum products. This also led to a devaluing of the regional differences in scents, of the origin of the incense and perfume plants, and took away a livelihood of traditional farmers who once cultivated these scents. The first "modern" perfume that used synthetics was called Jicky, and it hit the market in 1889. At first perfumers were cautious about the use of synthetics, because they knew they could not capture the depth, complexity, and beauty of natural scents. The newly created synthetics were, according to Mandy Aftel, a natural perfumer and author of the book *Essence and Alchemy,* "an oxymoron, utilitarian components of a luxurious, sensual product." However, as they began to be used, they started to dominate the blends, and become the icon for modernity (Aftel, 2001, p. 40).

A perfumer by the name of François Coty gave the modern perfume industry its other important new discovery. Coty opened his own perfume shop in 1908 in Paris, and along with the popularity of his first fragrance, La Rose Jacqueminot, he had created the first perfume packaged in small decorative bottles. Before this, perfumes were sold in apothecary bottles, and then when women brought them home they were transferred into decorative bottles. This new invention made perfume more accessible and easy to use for the individual. (Aftel, 2001).

The most bold and adventurous use of the new synthetics came with the development of Chanel No. 5. This synthetic was a derivative of an aldehyde, which at that time was the new chemical compound class for synthetics. Chanel No. 5 was thought of as creative because it did not try to copy naturals, and it was not formulated with the normal concepts of perfumery (Aftel, 2001).

The contemporary perfumes that have come to be are mostly linear in formulation. They are designed to produce a "punch" to your senses all at once, and then fade. They are not like the naturals that were complex and deep, offering a mystery to the senses of the beholder. They don't mix with the wearer's body chemistry, or change with time on the skin, as do the natural scents (Aftel, 2001).

The Environmental Protection Agency (EPA) has confirmed that poor air quality can cause neurological and physical problems such as headaches, dizziness, fatigue, and forgetfulness, so why is it we have not seen the connection of the prolific use of synthetics with our health? About 80 to 90 percent of synthetic fragrances are petroleum products that volatilize into the air to reach our nostrils, and they also can linger on our clothing and surroundings for months. Some synthetic perfumes are also known to be neurotoxins (Williams, 2004).

Today our sense of smell has become deadened by the overuse of these synthetic scents in the wide variety of products we are faced with every day. They are in our foods, our environment, in the cleansers we bathe our skin and households with, and the list goes on. It is almost difficult to smell a natural scent and not think of a product, such as lemons and wood polish, anymore. It is no wonder that incense has not been immune to this phenomena, and no wonder why the vast majority of incense is chalked full of synthetic fragrance. However, as incense is not a utilitarian product, why would we deprive ourselves of the beauty of natural scents? Why not worship with a product that honors nature, spirituality, and has the potential to add to the livelihoods of rural people around the globe? Why not get back to the real pleasure and appreciation of natural incense?

HOW THE SENSE OF SMELL WORKS

Each time we inhale, we also smell. Our noses are equipped with small, dime-sized patches of olfactory membranes that supply the nerve endings to signal to our brains the sense of smell. We have hundreds of millions of these olfactory nerve cells, and each one has about six to twelve hairs, or cilia, with receptors. These nerve cells are each replaced every twenty-eight days. Every odor molecule fits into a specific receptor cell. As the receptors are stimulated by odors that are brought in by our inhalations, the nerve cells fire and send signals to the brain. The area of the brain that then processes the sense of smell is the oldest part of the brain, the limbic lobe, which is associated with our deepest desires and impulses, sexual and emotional impulses, including fear, joy, anxiety, depression, and anger. The limbic system also has direct control of the heart rate, blood pressure, breathing, stress levels, hormone balance, and memory (Williams, 2004; Aftel, 2001).

The sense of smell is the only one of our five senses to be connected directly to the brain, and the olfactory membranes are the only places in the body where the central nervous system comes into direct contact with the environment. Our other senses all go through the thalamus first, which acts as a switchboard operator for the brain. The thalamus sends the impulses on to other areas of the brain, including the cerebral cortex. When an odor molecule stimulates a nerve cell lining, an electrical impulse is then sent to the olfactory bulb, which then transmits impulses to the gustatory center (where tastes are perceived), the amygdala (where emotional memories are stored), and other parts of the limbic center of the brain. This is why a whiff alone of one scent can elicit deep emotions in us, even before we have perceived them consciously (Aftel, 2001; Williams, 2004).

The limbic lobe consists of certain brain centers, one of them being the hippocampus. Since the hippocampus has the ability to directly stimulate the hypothalamus, it may enhance hormonal functions. The hypothalamus is our hormonal control center in the brain, producing important hormones as growth hormones, sex hormones, and neurotransmitters such as serotonin. Since scents may cause reactions in the limbic lobe through the hippocampus to activate the hypothalamus, it can be seen how they may exert physiological changes in the body. This is much of the basis of the therapeutic use of essential oils, and may explain some of the therapeutic activity of medicinal incense (Williams, 2004).

In an evolutionary viewpoint, it may make some sense about why our sense of smell has become so weakened compared to other, "less evolved" creatures. When we walked on all fours, our sense of smell was close to the ground, our environment, each other's genitals, and to scent trails that we relied upon. However, as we began to walk more upright, we lost proximity to those things, and so our olfactory membranes were not needed as much. This is when our other senses became more important for gaining access to information of the world (Aftel, 2001).

As explained earlier, the sense of smell has also lost its importance at least in a cultural viewpoint. This occurred around the time of the Enlightenment, when the sense of sight and science became dominant. However we know that our sense of smell can be trained and made keener, as there are numerous examples of people, such as Helen Keller, who developed a strong sense of smell when their other senses are compromised. Have you ever wondered why we say, "I would have to see that with my own two eyes to believe it?" Most of us have lost touch with our own sense of smell so much, that if our eyes are closed we could not tell what the item was that we were smelling.

The sense of smell is far from history, however. It is an area of science that, although not a popular, still holds many mysteries yet to be discovered. One misconception is that scent is just a sensation in our bodies that is produced by the scent molecules interacting with our receptors. On the contrary, it has been shown that scent can actually enter the blood stream, and therefore presumably produce biochemical interactions. For example, after mice inhaled sandalwood oil, the sandalwood derivatives alpha-santalol (6.1 ng/ml), beta-santalol (5.3 ng/ml), and alpha-santalene (0.5 ng/ml) could be found in the blood samples of the mice. Likewise, when they inhaled the pure fragrance compounds that are present in so many plants, coumarin and alpha-terpineol, these compounds were also present in the blood samples (at 7.7 ng/nl, and 6.9 ng/ml, respectively). It is also well documented that inhalations of fragrance through the nose goes to the brain, where it has neurological effects that may alter blood pressure, pulse, and mood, and it may also have sedative effects. Perhaps the early belief that the sense of smell could directly alter our health was not so far-fetched (Jirovetz et al., 1992; Williams, 2004).

THE LINK BETWEEN TASTE AND SCENT

Tastes are generally divided into five qualities: salty, sweet, sour, bitter, and umami (the flavor of glutamate). The qualities of smells, on the other hand, have never been agreed upon. As discussed in the beginning of the chapter, the sense of smell is the one sense that seems to have no words that are able to describe it. The best we have been able to come up with is to describe it through our other senses, especially our sense of taste. Even the great philosophers were in a state of disagreement, whereas Plato divided smells into pleasant and unpleasant, Aristotle classified them into seven subclasses. Linnaeus, in the eighteenth century delineated smells into seven different types: aromatic, fragrant, alliaceous (garlic), ambrosial (musky), hircinous (goaty), repulsive, and nauseous. Added to this list later were ethereal (fruity) and empyreumatic (roasted coffee).

A lot of what we perceive as taste, however, is in fact olfaction. Accordingly, when we perceive a defect in our taste—as when we have a cold and a stuffy nose and our food does not taste as good as usual—it is in fact only a defect in our ability to smell. Olfaction alters flavor. The perception of food flavor is made up of different aspects of foods: the smell, taste, texture, and temperature, smell being very important. Disorders of taste and smell have been difficult to treat conventionally, since there has been little understanding and knowledge of how these senses work. In fact, alterations in taste or smell can be a signal that some other disease process is at work in the body. Approximately 2.7 million American adults have difficulty or decreased sense of smell, whereas approximately 1.1 million have problems with their sense of taste. Deficiencies in the senses of taste and smell can cause anxiety, depression, and even nutritional deficiencies because people may eat less. Since taste is such an important sense in experiencing life and socializing, it holds a place next to smell in how our early memories are shaped and remembered (Ackerman, 1990).

Taste is also known as the social sense. Humans rarely choose to dine alone, as much of the enjoyment of the sense of taste is social enjoyment. It is also the reason that the act of eating meals together is so important for family bonding. It is as if it is a social contract that brings us together by "breaking bread." All of our holidays are associated with eventful meals, as are important moments in our lives, such as weddings. Taste and the act of eating is also ritualized in certain religions, such as taking communion for Catholics, or the act of eating horseradish by Jews at seder to symbolize the tears shed by their ancestors.

As with the sense of smell, the sense of taste has much to do about how we enjoy the "richness" of life. Without either of these senses, life becomes dull, and people are prone to depression and anxiety. Incense, as with food, is used to mark special rites of passage and holidays. It is one of the rituals that bring us more richness to the experiences with which we use it.

SCENT AND MEMORY

In the beginning of this chapter you may have imagined some of your favorite smells and the memories that are attached to them. You may have remembered how your lover's shirt brings a memory so close to your mind that you feel instantly close to him or her, or perhaps you remembered the smell of a certain food that instantly transported you to your parent's house. We have all experienced the powerful link between scent and memory, and how scent acts as our magical time machine that can instantly transport us to distant memories and make us relive them as if we were there—with all the feelings attached to that experience intact. Part of the explanation of how scent is able to do this has been discussed in explaining how the sense of smell works.

Our sense of smell is the only sense that is directly linked to the brain—to the limbic lobe, a part of the brain responsible for our deepest desires and emotions. As it is the only sense that is not processed in the thalamus first, it is the reason we can be transported to these places in our memory before we consciously even know we are smelling a scent.

The sense of smell is among the first senses to awaken when we are babies—it guides us to the smell of our mother's milk, and we can differentiate our mothers from others just by the sense of smell alone. Babies smile when they smell the scent of their mothers, and this in turn pleases the mother. These are some of our earliest fond memories that the sense of smell evokes in us (Aftel, 2001).

The sense of smell is also important to us when we are adults, as it can alter our learning and ability to do certain tasks. Research has confirmed that certain aromas are associated with enhanced task performance. For example, in one study, peppermint odor was investigated for its effect on work performance, measured by typing performance, memorization, and alphabetization. When the protocol was followed with the peppermint odor, there was a significant improvement in performance, measured by differences in the gross speed, net speed, and accuracy of the typing task. Alphabetization also improved strongly when in the presence of the peppermint odor. The researchers concluded that peppermint was associated with a general arousal of attention, enabling the participants to be more focused on their tasks and increase performance (Barker et al., 2003).

Lavender and rosemary, according to essential oil therapy theory, have somewhat opposite actions to each other: lavender is supposed to be calming and help you to relax, and rosemary is supposed to be stimulating. For many years, essential oil therapy was laughed at as hocus pocus by the scientific community (and largely still is), but recently an increasing number of clinical studies are confirming its therapeutic effects. In several studies, lavender has indeed been confirmed to have a calming effect, and to be able to lower people's response to stress. In another study, lavender and rosemary were studied for their effect on cognition and mood. In this randomized study, rosemary stimulated the memory and also increased performance, whereas lavender did the opposite. Lavender and rosemary also produced a feeling of contentment that was significantly higher than the control group that was subjected to no scent (Moss et al., 2003).

In a study on the effect of essential oils on brain activity, subjects' EEG (electroencephalogram) changes were monitored directly after inhalation of essential oils. Four odors—lavender, chamomile, sandalwood, and eugenol—were applied to the subjects, and then both a subjective evaluation and EEG changes were monitored. From the twenty-two adjective pairs that were used to describe the sensory experience by the subjects, four basic factors were described: "comfortable feeling," "cheerful feeling," "natural feeling," and "feminine feeling." The scents that were used to describe "comfortable feeling" were ranked highest to lowest in producing that feeling: lavender, eugenol, chamomile, and sandalwood. The alpha 1 (8 to 10 Hz) of EEG at the parietal and posterior temporal regions significantly decreased after inhalation of lavender, as well as after inhalation of eugenol and chamomile. The researchers linked lower alpha 1 brain activity to the subjective feeling of being comfortable (Masago et al., 2000).

These have been just a few of the clinical studies that have been performed recently in discovering how exactly scent interacts with the brain, memory, and our health. As the research mounts, scents will be sure to play an increasing role in our lives as lifestyle, therapeutic, and performance aids.

SCENT AS A DIRECT PATH TO THE SOUL

The sense of smell has been described as being able to detect the "savor of life." In a description of one man's experience after completely losing his sense of smell, he said it was like life lost its savor. There was suddenly no depth to life, and all the things that he had taken for granted smelling before, such as books, people, the city, and spring were sorely missed. It is as though scent gives depth or soul to those very objects that surround us every day. Without it life seems more lifeless and it is more difficult to enjoy (Classen et al., 1994).

Because scent gives depth and soul to everything around us, it also touches us physically, emotionally, and often spiritually. There is no better example of scents that touch us on a spiritual level than incense. Although this is difficult to prove or even define (how something could affect us on a spiritual level), there seems to be no coincidence that incense is used in different and disconnected religions and spirituality across the globe. Perhaps it has to do with the anatomy of the sense of smell, and how this sense is processed in the oldest part of the brain, and in a sense in the most ancient part of ourselves. Since the limbic lobe of the brain is also the seat of the emotions and sexual impulses, it may be the most connected to our sense of what it feels to be human and to possess a soul.

Through his book *Phantoms in the Brain,* noted neurologist V.S. Ramachandran stirred up all kinds of controversy about the role of the brain in our perception and experiencing God. One of the chapters is dedicated to the phenomenon of intense religious experiences by people with some types of injuries in the temporal lobe of the brain. Whereas some church leaders have claimed that he has uncovered some sort of God antennae in the brain, atheists have also used his research as proof that God does not exist (Ramachandran, 1999).

One way to understand the connection between scents and the soul is to examine the effect of scents on meditation. Certain scents make us more able to relax, while others may help us to focus. Others are said to be able to open up the mind and the soul in meditation and to spiritual experiences. Certain scents in the form of incense have been used to deepen meditation, and in this way to deepen us into what it is to be ourselves. Meditation can bring us the understanding of what it is to be our true selves, and through this understanding we are able to dissipate much of the suffering that accompanies life.

However, deepening our sense of smell beyond its use in meditation or in using smells therapeutically has a role. Smells can help us live more content, relaxed, and stress-free lives, as well as bring richer meaning to life. To develop our sense of smell more keenly and awaken to the world of scents and their complexities around us is to awaken to what it means to be more alive.

PERFUME AND FRAGRANCE ALLERGIES AND SENSITIVITIES

Some people are overly sensitive to scents, and their inhalation can give them headaches and dizziness, whereas for other people even strong scents go unnoticed. Sensitivities to scents may also cause someone to get puffy-eyed and break out into hives when they come into contact with these fragrances. Many other symptoms are reported with fragrance allergies, including nausea, fatigue, shortness of breath, difficulty with concentration, respiratory complaints, allergies, and perhaps even asthma. Although some people enjoy fragranced products, a growing number of people are saying "enough is enough!"

These sensitivities to perfumes and fragrances are not just "made up," however, since some perfumes have been confirmed to be neurotoxins. Some perfumes have been linked to central nervous system disorders, headaches, confusion, dizziness, short-term memory loss, anxiety, depression, disorientation, and mood swings. In addition, contact dermatitis to fragrances is one of the most commonly reported symptoms of perfume allergies. Multiple chemical sensitivity (MCS), a health condition in which exposure to one chemical causes sensitivities to other chemicals, can be particularly disabling because often fragrances are so abundant in our environment that those who suffer from MCS can barely go outside (Williams, 2004).

Fragrance allergies and sensitivities are a growing public health problem. More than 5,000 different fragrances are formulated in products that are used daily, including soaps, beauty aids, household cleaners, laundry aids, drugs, foods, paper and plastic products, industrial greases, and solvents. Moreover, items that are labeled "unscented" or "fragrance free" are not always what they claim to be. It has come to the point where some high schools, public attractions, and public buildings have posted policies of no fragrance use by their inhabitants (Williams, 2004).

One type of synthetic fragrance, the chemical AETT (acetylethyltetramethyletetralin), which was used in a number of personal care products, became such a public health concern that it was withdrawn by the perfume and fragrance industry. Despite evidence in a number of animal studies that it could cause significant brain and spinal cord damage, the U.S. Food and Drug Administration (FDA) in the 1970s refused to ban it. Luckily it was withdrawn from the market by the industry, but only after public concern had mounted (Eiermann, 1980; Spencer et al., 1979). Another synthetic fragrance, 6-MC (6-methylcoumarin), was found to be a photocontact allergen. One study on individuals with a history for having photosensitivity reactions found that the incidence of the photocontact allergies has been declining, possibly due to industry and consumers' increased awareness and preference for products without photoallerginic ingredients. However, the incidence of photosensitivity by people using sunscreens with these agents included is increasing. Overall, fragrances are the leading cause of allergic contact dermatitis due to their inclusion in cosmetics, with photosensitivities being less common. (DeLeo et al., 1992; Larsen, 1985; Williams, 2004).

As some people have begun to turn their backs on products containing synthetic fragrances, the industry has responded by creating "unscented" or "fragrance-free" products. However, these products may still contain fragrance chemicals that are used to cover the scent of other chemicals in the product. In fact, when a fragrance is used in a product, the companies are not even required by law to disclose what kind of fragrance has been used because many companies claim these are trade secrets. All that is required is that they list the word "fragrance" on the label if it is added. It has gotten to the point that synthetic fragrances are almost unavoidable in this culture (Williams, 2004).

Common scented or synthetic products that cause sensitivities are gasoline, diesel exhaust, acetone, fabric softeners, scented laundry detergents, acetate (often in hairspray), nail polish paints, magic markers, carpet solvents, deodorized cat litter, scented shampoos and conditioners, propane/butane, cigarette smoke, bug spray, furniture polish, and mothballs. The FDA has a program in place for reporting adverse reactions to cosmetics, and through this program, an increased number of adverse reactions to fragrances in products such as these are being reported from fragrance compounds (Williams, 2004).[1]

Prior to all the allergies, illnesses, and backlash to fragrances because of the use of synthetic scents, natural scents and essences were used for millennia for healing purposes. Among these was incense. Incense has played an important role in traditional medicines of many distinct cultures since the beginning of time for man.

ESSENTIAL OILS AND FLOWER ESSENCES FOR HEALING

Essential oils are the volatile components of plants—including flowers, fruits, seeds, leaves, bark, stems, and roots—that during distillation are separated first (see Photo 2.2). In any essential oil may be hundreds of different chemical compounds, and the profile of the essential oil may be altered by numerous factors, including the part of

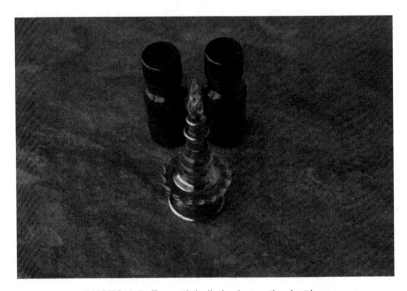

PHOTO 2.2. Essential oils in decorative bottles.

plant it was extracted from, the plant chemotype, and the growing conditions, such as soil, geographical region, altitude, water, climate, harvest and postharvest handling, season, and the process of distillation. Essential oils are used for numerous applications, including cosmetic, flavor and fragrance, and therapeutics, and it is important that when an essential oil is used for internal use, it is a therapeutic grade that does not contain harmful solvents. Adulterated essential oils, and synthetic oils that are disguised as essential oils are, unfortunately, common and caution should be exercised when choosing essential oil sources to consume.

Essential oils differ greatly from synthetic fragrances, one of the most important ways being that they are made up of many—often hundreds—of different natural chemical components. With the complexity of the essential oils, a built-in safety factor is thought to exist in that whereas one component alone may exert a strong and undesirable effect, the other components mixed in the essential oil that may counteract these effects, or at least dilute them. Synthetic fragrances, on the other hand, are composed of just one chemical. This is similar to the common argument for the safety of herbal medicine versus pharmaceuticals. Whereas a single pharmaceutical is designed to have one particular action and is strong and disrupts the body's homeostasis, an herbal medicine often contains many components that result in a more balanced effect.

In order to prevent confusion between inferior or adulterated oils in Europe, a set of standards have been developed called AFNOR (Association of French Normalization Organization Regulation) and ISO (International Standards Organization). Essential oils are certified by both AFNOR and ISO standards only if they are both high quality and have the characteristic profile of chemical components for that oil. In order to deliver high-quality products in the United States, some U.S.–based companies aim to comply with these standards.

Beyond the quality of the oil itself, it is important to buy products that are as safe and natural as possible. Many companies have products—from dish soaps to shampoos—that sound like they have beneficial essential oils included, but the quality of the oils or the amount of the oils is often low and poor, and other fragrances are added to give the illusion that the essential oils are producing the characteristic odor of the product. In addition, if you are looking for a product that is "good for you," keep your eye on the other ingredients in the product and make sure that you are not duped into buying a largely synthetic and potentially harmful product when you wanted something natural and beneficial (Williams, 2004).

Essential oils are important in the understanding of incense because part of the characteristic scent emitted when a plant is burned, such as incense, is volatile oil, or essential oils. Essential oils are also added to some incense products, such as sticks and cones. As with other products claiming to be natural and contain essential oil, it is important to know if other synthetic fragrances have been added to an incense product.

As explained earlier, because the limbic lobe of the brain contains the hippocampus, which can activate the hypothalamus—our hormonal production center—the use of essential oils therapeutically (as well as incense) can be seen to have some scientific basis. Indeed, preliminary research on essential oils have found them to be able to alter energy levels, help reduce stress and trauma, and even to stimulate growth hormone, which may enhance our longevity and youthfulness. Dr. Alan Hirsch of the Smell and Taste Treatment Center and Research Foundation in Chicago (cited in Williams, 2004) believes smells can alter the mood faster than anything else. However, as we have begun to understand the positive effects of essential oils on mood and well-being, we still know very little about the effect of synthetic fragrance on us (Williams, 2004).

Another way that essential oils have been found to exert a therapeutic effect is through enhancing the brain's level of oxygen. Research has found that the sesquiterpenes present in sandalwood, frankincense, *Melissa,* myrrh, and clove oils can increase oxygen levels in the brain by 28 percent, which undoubtedly may produce other benefits in the body. The benefit of the increased oxygen is the increase in the activity of the hypothalamus and its subsequent effect on emotions, learning, and attitude. Other benefits include improving immune function, hormone balance, and energy levels (Williams, 2004).

Hirsch has also found certain essential oils to have effects on weight loss, satiety, and libido. In one study, peppermint essential oil was given to participants who had tried and failed other weight loss measures. The study involved more than 3,000 participants over six months, and found that the average weight loss with the use of peppermint was over five pounds monthly. In a separate study on the effects of different essential oils on libido, thirty-one men were tested in a double-blind, randomized design. The scents that produced the largest increase in libido were a combination of lavender and pumpkin (Williams, 2004).

Many other clinical studies are mounting on the therapeutic effects of essential oils. For example, aroma inhalation via an aroma lamp (containing lavender, peppermint, rosemary and clary sage) was tested on nursing students for its effect on students' stress levels. The aromas resulted in lower anxiety and perceived stress scores, and fewer physical symptoms being experienced by the students (Park and Lee, 2004). In another study, the perception of pain caused by heat, pressure, and ischemic pain was found to be lower after treatment with lavender and rosemary essential oils (Gedney et al., 2004).

Essential oils are also being researched and have been found to be good as adjunct treatments for certain diseases and conditions. In one study, the use of lavender tincture was compared to a common pharmaceutical treatment for depression, imipramine. Although lavender alone did not provide as good therapeutic efficacy as imipramine, when the two were combined, the result was a higher efficacy than using the imipramine alone. The authors suggested that the lavender tincture may be of benefit for treating mild to moderate depression (Akhondzadeh et al., 2003).

In the early 1900s a physician named Edward Bach developed a branch of homeopathic or herbal medicine using only flower extracts as ingredients. His belief was that in order for a patient to improve his or her condition and heal, the patient must improve his or her emotional condition first. Flower essences are dilute extracts of various types of flowers, and today they are made in several different lines and companies beyond Bach Flower Essences. Although not much research exists to confirm their efficaciousness, they continue to be a safe and popular form of alternative medicine. Perhaps there is some correlation to the efficacy of incense (those made from flowers) and the efficacy of flower essence therapy.

INCENSE FOR KEEPING TIME

Incense and the sense of smell has also helped us to perceive and measure time. This is because historically incense was used in the Far

East and East Asian countries as a means of keeping time. The first time-keeping devices that all civilizations have developed seems to be some derivative form of the sundial, ranging in its most primitive state being a tree or pole erected in a cleared area, to its more developed form of intricate gold sundials. The second known form of keeping time seems to be the clepsydra, or water clock, and the third the use of incense burning to keep time. For centuries these three forms of time measurement were the only methods that were used, until the much later advent of the mechanical clock. Time measurement began as something that could be perceived mostly by the sense of sight, as sundials and water clocks need to be viewed in order to interpret the time. The sense of touch was used later, after the advent of the mechanical clock for blind persons to know the time, and at one time—though it was never widely used—there was even a clock that employed the sense of taste! The sense of smell was used since the earliest times to measure time in the form of incense in the countries of the Far East, and these practices were adopted throughout Asia (Bedini, 1994).

Incense was probably chosen for time measurement due to its constant burning time and its common use in the home and in worship in those days. Incense burning was among humanity's common experiences, and it became an activity that was so common that everyone knew approximately how long it took to burn a stick of incense, as did other common activities such as drinking a cup of tea or eating a bowl of rice. In fact, "the time of burning an incense stick" *(i chu hsianghsiag ti shih hou)* is repeated in ancient Chinese writings and poems referring to the passage of a specific amount of time (Bedini, 1994).

The incense used to keep time first began as incense sticks. These were essentially joss sticks (see Photo 2.3) that had time measurement markings on them usually in two-hour blocks. Before incense, the sundial, the water clock, and other primitive means of keeping time—such as looking in a cat's eyes—were used, but only incense survived until modern times. This is probably because incense held more meaning and has been a welcome part of people's lives since ancient times. For example, incense was believed to be able to maintain a pleasant state of mind, sustain the spirit, and attract auspicious gods—not to mention lovers—to oneself. For these reasons, it was used in all sorts of common daily activities, and also in civil (as in the

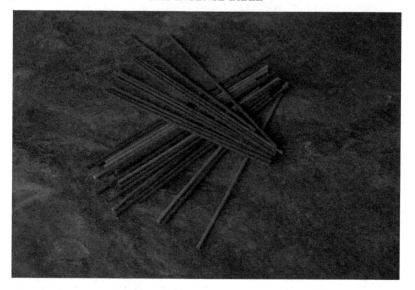

PHOTO 2.3. Joss sticks.

civil offices) and formal affairs, such as in the presence of the emperor (Bedini, 1994).

Incense was used not only for time, but also for other time-measurement activities, such as in the measurement of water. The water measured would be the amount that flowed in the time it took for incense to burn. Another activity that incense was used for was to time an imperial progression, which was always aligned with the most beneficial astrological timing. Among the poorest classes, a knotted cord made of punk (a decayed woody material) was used as an incense time-keeping device. The spacing of the knots determined the time increments (Bedini, 1994).

Later, other incense devices were used for time measurement that replaced the incense stick, such as the dragon boat alarm, the incense spiral, and the incense seal. The dragon boat alarm was a model replica of a boat that had at its bow and stern the head and the tail of the dragon, respectively. Along the hull of the boat were wires that were placed in order to hold an incense stick, and then lying over top of the incense stick in specified increments were silk threads that had bells attached to each end. When the burning of the incense stick reached the thread, the thread would break and release the bells into the hull, making an alarming sound. This would notify someone that a certain time had passed (Bedini, 1994).

Spiral incense coils were used to keep time when the time passage that needed measuring was too long for an incense stick. For example, the coils were used during night watches in order for different shifts to replace one another. Today coils are used as insect repellents in homes and as offerings in Buddhist temples, especially prevalent in Southeast Asia, where they are suspended from the ceiling rafters. These coils have also started to appear on the market in the United States, in such popular shops as the Pottery Barn, as they have a distinct and decorative look in the home and garden (Bedini, 1994).

The use of the incense seal came from a sect of Buddhism called tantra. In one of the tantric scriptures, a feature of one of these tantric rituals was titled, "The [Incense] Seal of Avalokitésvara Bodhisatt-va." The text detailed the burning of a trail of incense in the shape of a Siddham seal character, and with that certain spiritual meanings were to come (see Chapter 3). After the translation of this tantric text into Chinese, the Chinese came up with a system of using the seal not only for prayer, but also for time telling. Since the Buddhist services were performed six times daily, the seal was used as a means for dividing time. Later, the incense seal became commonplace outside of the temples in civil life as a means for keeping time, and different adaptations of the seals were made (Bedini, 1994).

THE DIVINITY OF SCENTS

Scents are often referred to as essences or spirits. They are somewhere between the physical and metaphysical worlds, giving them a powerful effect on the mind and body. Mandy Aftel (2001) describes scents to be "at once holy and carnal, spiritual and material, arcane and modern, tangible and intangible, profound and superficial."

According to Classen (Aftel, 2001, p. 18),

> The common association of odor with breath and with the life-force makes smell a source of elemental power, and therefore an appropriate symbol and medium for divine life and power. Odors can strongly attract or repel, rendering them forceful metaphors for good and evil. Odors are also ethereal, they cannot be grasped or retained; in their elusiveness they convey a sense of both the

mysterious presence and the mysterious absence of God. Finally, odors are ineffable, they transcend our ability to define them through language, as religious experience is said to do.

Before the use of scents for making perfumes and scented oils and unguents, scents were used in spiritual rituals across the world. The reasons it was included in these rituals vary, and many overlap, including as a means of purification, to communicate or call spirits, to chase spirits away, as a means of inspiration and deepening meditation, and transport of the soul. In fact, it is interesting to look at the Latin bases of the words *perfume* and *incense*. Perfume means literally "through smoke" *(per fumum)*, and incense means literally "something burnt" *(incensum)*.

Scents in worship have also been prepared in other ways, one of the next oldest being as anointing oils, such as fragrant oils and unguents. Many more indigenous cultures use fragrant oils and scents on their bodies in such as way, and this has also been traced back to the time of the Egyptians. The Egyptians had a fragrant blend called kyphi that was used in many ways, and for many purposes. Kyphi was said to be cleansing, have a calming effect, induce dreaming, sweeten the breath, restore the imagination, and to induce sleep. In early Christian tradition, the use of an anointing oil called chrism, a consecrated oil, began. Chrism is still used today for priests and kings, and in fact the same blend continues to be used for anointing the King of England—a mixture of rose, orange blossom, jasmine, cinnamon, benzoin, civet, musk, ambergris, and sesame oil (Aftel, 2001).

The use of incense and anointing oils was for purposes that often served the mind, body, and spirit. In ancient times, and in other non-Western cultures today, the separation of mind, body, and spirit was never as great as it is today. Instead of treating the mind, body, and spirit as three distinct areas, with distinct concepts about what affects them, they were thought of as all truly connected.

In Egypt, as in many more indigenous cultures, where the doctors were also priests and the "practice" of medicine overlapped strongly into spiritual realms, the use of scented oils, incense, and other preparations were used heavily. Later in pre-Western civilization, the use of these scented materials was spread among several groups of people, the occultists, the perfumers, religious/spiritual practitioners, and the physicians. Occultists still used aromatics in similar ways to their pagan predecessors into the sixteenth and seventeenth centuries.

Incense symbolized many things in spiritual terms. As previously mentioned, in some cultures, such as the ancient Romans and early Christians, incense symbolized the odor of God or the gods, and such a scent on its own could indicate a god's presence or holiness. The grace, holiness, and loveliness of the divine was thought to exude a sweet smell. This sweet smell could be embodied by living people, such as saints, called the odor of sanctity, and it has been noted in certain righteous individuals in history, as it was said to be present at the death of Sir Lancelot (Aftel, 2001). The Buddhists of China and Japan thought incense smoke to literally be the teachings of Buddha, and because of this they referred to the practice as "listening" to the incense, as many still do today.

Sweet scents were also symbolic of paradise, or the Garden of Eden. Many references have been made to the overwhelming sweet and voluptuous odors present in the Garden of Eden, and at times scents were used to re-create this paradise. That many types of incenses, including frankincense and myrrh, came from areas near where the Garden of Eden was thought to be located gives credence to this idea (Fischer-Rizzi, 1996).

As synthetics became popular, the use of natural aromatics faded away greatly from religious practice. Those who perform ceremonies, be they Buddhist or Catholic priests, often buy mass-produced, spiritual/religious blends, such as the "Three Kings Blend," or "Temple Blend," and they are unaware, and sometimes largely uncaring, that these blends might contain synthetics. What would our spiritual practices look like if we really cared about what incenses we used, and what kind of connection to these scents might we uncover through reintroducing them to our practice? Perhaps a greater sense of awareness and enjoyment of the world might be gained by our re-developed sense of smell if we brought the association of divine or spiritual ecstasy to the natural sweet smells that surround us daily.

NOTE

1. The numbers for consumers to report adverse reactions by fragrance or other chemicals in cosmetic or body care products are (800) 535-4555 (nonemergency), (301) 443-1240 (emergency), or (888) 463-6332 (for product information).

Chapter 3

The Pervasiveness of Incense

In every house, boat, street and garden the traveler, after a little observation beholds signs of religious import, principally in the innumerable joss sticks that are forever smoking . . . through cities and villages; in enormous temples . . . and on barren crags by the salt sea . . . and in the hut of the beggar . . . appear the silent but everlasting signs of adoration.

Written by a nineteenth-century American observer in China
(Bedini, 1994)

Imagine tiny spirals of smoke rising from every continent of the globe. Then try to observe numerous rituals, chants, meditations in complete silence, and prayers that ride those tiny spirals into the heavens. Perhaps God waits to hear these prayers on a highway of scent, or maybe spirits gobble up the incense as soon as it is lit. Perhaps all the good spirits or angels come to see as the bad ones flee. Or maybe the incense smoke washes over the supplicants like water cleansing them of impurities. Incense use is so pervasive throughout the globe, cultures, and time that only snapshots of how people use it and view it and little pearls of wisdom can tell its story.

THE EARLY INCENSE TRAIL IN EGYPTIAN, GREEK, AND ROMAN TIMES

It is thought that incense was first used in the countries of the Near East, such as Egypt, and then traveled to India in an early period, and then on to other Asian and European countries from there. Incense use in Egypt is known from as far back as the eighth century, when the Egyptians had a highly evolved relationship with aromatics. They obtained the juice from certain succulent flowers and plants, the pulp of fruits, resins and gums from trees, oily substances from seeds, and mixed them with spices, wine, honey, and oils to develop their blends for incense and unguents (Aftel, 2001).

In the earliest times of the Greeks, incense or fragrant oils were not used. *The Iliad* describes the early Greeks as brutal savages who had no refined sense of smell and who did not use incense in burial rites. Later, in *The Odyssey,* came mention of perfumed robes as well as the burning of cedar wood for the scent. In the sixth and seventh centuries, as the Greeks developed closer relationships with Syria and Egypt, they also developed more luxuries and civilization and began to import perfumes and incenses (Atchley, 1909).

The gods of Greek and Roman times were routinely offered incense as a sacrifice. The gods of this time were thought to reside in a fragrant Mount Olympus, and to be fond of similar sweet scents as we humans were. For this reason, fragrant incense, flowers, and perfume were offered in rituals. The Romans applied aromatics lavishly to statues of sacred icons, as perfumes for their own bodies, on walls, horses, and even dogs (Classen et al., 1994).

The gods of these times were also thought to be fond of burnt animal flesh, and this was offered after sacrificial killings. Along with the sacrifice and burning of all kinds of animals, incense was always burned. However, incense was offered alone as well. The Pythagorean cult that originated in the sixth century BC did not believe in the sacrifice of animals, as they thought it cruel, and instead believed incense to be a better offering (Classen et al., 1994; Atchley, 1909).

In some cultures, such as the Roman and Egyptian cultures, it was believed that sweet fragrances were needed in order to assist the soul in separating from the body after death so it may ascend to the spirit realm. For this reason, the Egyptians had elaborate methods for fragrancing the body—both inside and out—and the Romans would pour or burn aromatics over the ashes of the dead (Aftel, 2001).

More references to the use of incense in rituals were described as the Greek civilization advanced. The festival of Hera, called Daedala, was a time of great offerings of wine and incense. In addition, whenever anyone consulted th oracle of the Temple of Ceres at Patras, the priestess would pray, offer incense, and then look down a sacred well with a mirror where the answer was said to be seen. In the Orphic

Hymns, different fragrant substances were associated with different gods—frankincense was for one, saffron for another, myrrh yet for another (Atchley, 1909).

The Romans basically believed in the humoral theory, in which the basic building blocks of the world were composed of cold, wet, dry, and hot qualities. In this way they believed the sweet and spicy scents such as those of incense to be of the hot and dry qualities, whereas foul scents were associated with cold and wet qualities. This made sense then to them that many of the aromatics used at those times, such as frankincense and myrrh, were from the hot dry regions of Arabia (Classen et al., 1994).

This belief that smells were part of the world in a very basic level may have led to further connotations between the sense of smell and intelligence, as being able to keenly perceive smell was recognized as a sign of intelligence. The Latin word *sagax*(and our word *sagacious*) demonstrates this because it was used to not only mean a keen sense of smell, but also that someone was intelligent and clever. Indeed, the very act of emitting and inhaling odor was correlated with the process of attaining knowledge. This is an interesting belief when compared to the Japanese Buddhist concept of "listening to the incense" in order to gain the teachings of Buddha, as I will discuss later (Classen et al., 1994).

In Roman times incense was burned before the statues of gods during procession, and were left either in doorways along the procession route or carried by hand. Incense was even a part of the Circensian games, which included a procession of dancers and musicians followed by people carrying gold and silver censers with various religious and civil signs inscribed on them, followed by people carrying the images of gods. In the procession for the goddess Isis, a large number of people carried candles and torches, while priests carried lanterns and an altar. At the head of the procession were women who wore garlands of flowers, and people who strewed herbs, balm, and other fragrant substances (Atchley, 1909).

In earlier Roman times, it was not customary to burn the dead but to bury them. However, before the burial the body was washed and anointed. Later it became customary for the bodies of the dead to be cremated, and in some instances large quantities of incense and other spices were brought to the cremations. There is one story of a cremation in which large statues of frankincense and cinnamon were created of the departed and then burned on the pyre (Atchley, 1909).

ARABIAN SECRETS

The ancient trade routes of frankincense and myrrh were traveled by camel and kept secret from outsiders. The exact location of where frankincense and myrrh trees grew was surrounded by so much myth and secrecy that the outside world had no access to these trees. In the ancient land of Sheba—what is today Yemen and Oman—is the place where frankincense and myrrh trees originated. They grew only in the hot, stony, and lime-enriched desert belt that was protected from wind by the mountains. This was also native territory for other incense plants—such as balsam and cinnamon—all of which made the inhabitants of the Arabian region very wealthy. The beginning of the 2,200 mile trade route through the desert began in the town of Ma'rib, at the eastern corner of the foothills of Yemen. An oasis was located in the middle of the town, and large walls surrounded and protected it.

The Love of the Prophet

According to the prophet of Islam, Mohammed, he loved three things the most in this world: women, pleasant fragrances, and prayer. The most loved of the fragrances by Mohammed was musk. Musk comes from the scent gland of a deer, and when it is concentrated it smells of urine and ammonia, but when it is highly diluted it becomes an earthy and sensuous fragrance (Fischer-Rizzi, 1996). Yemeni women still use incense to perfume their clothing with musk, aloeswood, sandalwood, clove, and rose. Muslim women use an incense mixture called *bakhur,* which is made by the family to scent their *burkas* and *chadors*. The incense has a rose water and sugar base, and consists usually of the aforementioned incenses, as well as ground up conch shells called *duffer* (Hyams, 2004).

According to Muslim beliefs,

> As sweet scent is the nourishment of the spirit, and the spirit is the instrument of the faculties, and the faculties increase with scent; for it is beneficial for brain and heart and the other inter-

nal organs, and makes the heart rejoice, pleases the soul and re-vitalizes the spirit. (Hyams, 2004)

A close relationship is said to exist between scent and the good spirit, and scent is one of the most beloved things to the Prophet, who is held to be the most sweetly scented of all. It is believed that angels like sweet scents, and demons flee from them since they prefer only those scents that are putrid or foul smelling. In the *Sahih Muslim* from the Prophet, it is said that if someone offers you sweet-smelling plants, you are not to refuse them. Each region has a plant that is known as "the sweet-smelling plant" that is used in ritual and appreciated (Johnson, 1998).

In Muslim teachings sweet scents are thought to be able to enhance the preservation of health, to repel pain and suffering and their causes, and to strengthen the constitution. Sweet scents in the form of certain incenses or fumigants, such as aloeswood, may be further used to purify the essence of the air. The essence of the air is important according to the teachings of the Prophet because it is one of the six essential elements that is necessary for the preservation of the health of the body. Therefore, sweet scents in the form of incense are important for the well-being of mind and body in Muslim beliefs (Johnson, 1998).

When the temples of Arabia were built, musk was mixed in with the cement, and it is said that the odor of musk still is present thousands of years later. Adding to the sacred fragrance of the mosques is a rose water mixture that is sprayed. Today, because the musk deer is endangered, the seeds of the rose mallow functions as a substitute for musk (Fischer-Rizzi, 1996).

A number of other different scents and aromatic plants are used in Islamic rituals and festivities. During the twenty-seventh day of Ramadan—the celebratory feast for the birth of the prophet and the conclusion of fasting—one of the most intricate incense mixtures is used, which is comprised of sandalwood mixed with a number of other fragrant incenses. It is used to satisfy the negative energies that could appear during Ramadan (Fischer-Rizzi, 1996).

The Sufi Rose

The symbol of the Sufi came from a fragrant plant—the mystical rose—that was believed to be the "mother of all fragrances." Although many people think of the fragrance of rose to be that of romantic longing or desire, the Sufis connected it to the love of God, and the desire to be close to God. It was then used for this effect in incense burning mixtures.

The "father of all fragrances" was considered to be ambergris. However, the ambergris that the Sufi were fond of did not come from the sperm whale, which produces a substance more commonly called ambergris, but from trees, possibly *Pinus succinifera,* which is now extinct, or from other amber-producing trees. Ambergris creates a sweet, balsamic fragrance that is also believed to have healing qualities for the heart, including helping reduce anxiety, depression, and sadness.

The Sufi poets of the mystical order of Islam—Rumi, Hafiz, and Saadi—all used the sensual and emotion-stimulating praise of fragrances in their poetry. Avicenna, a famous physician and mystic, in his works, such as *The Canon of Medicine* (original title in Arabic: *"qanun fil tibb"*), described how fragrances were interrelated to the human soul, and the different conditions of the soul. He believed the soul of the plant was present in its fragrance, and that this could be called upon in the healing of human beings (Fischer-Rizzi, 1996).

INDIA'S BRIDGES TO INNER AWARENESS

It seems as if no other country possesses such a wealth of aromas as does India. A diversity of climatic zones—spanning the high elevations of the Himalayas down to the cape of the Indian Ocean—have enriched India with a diversity of aromatic plants. India is often thought of as the origin of many of the world's top incenses, as India was so influential in the spread of incense and Buddhism into Asian countries. The people of India use simple brass and stoneware incense burning vessels, as well as more ornate ones that may be created into the shapes of animals (usually in bronze) (Fischer-Rizzi, 1996).

In a visit of manufacturers of incense in Mysore, India, Christopher McMahon of White Lotus Aromatics found that prior to 1950 all the original companies of Mysore used all natural ingredients. Before this time India was rich in forest products that included spices, woods, herbs, roots, etc., that are used to make incense. The foundation of Indian culture, he explains, came from the belief of an unseen and powerful force that created the entire universe. This universe was seen to be composed of five basic elements: earth *(bhumi)*, fire *(ag)*, ether *(gaggan)*, air *(wayu)*, and water *(nir)*. The Supreme Power then gave these elements life, form, and expression by creating plants, animals, and the rest of the universe. The early people of India saw the universe in this way, and did not think of themselves as being the only conscious beings on earth. In order to find a way to express reverence and to listen to the other inhabitants of the world, they turned to nature to find something that could bring people close to the source of life, the Unseen Power. They sought some accessible medium that could transmit to people the unwritten and unspoken laws of true living. "Since most people could not spend so many years in deep meditation and contemplation as they (the leaders of the culture) had done, they needed to find outer symbols that could act as bridges to inner awareness," says McMahone (2001). It was the colorful and scented flora that was found to be able to so easily affect the heart and mind of any simple person, to bring them to a state of awareness that could open them for transformation. From this basic knowledge came teachings on life and a whole system of medicine that is Hindu-based, called Ayurveda, the "science of life" (McMahone, 2001).

In Ayurveda it was believed that illness stemmed from imbalances in a person's inner life. Early signs of imbalance often manifested in difficulty in the breathing pattern. It was found that reestablishing a good breathing pattern while inhaling the aroma of aromatic plants was a key to reestablishing balance and health. This is how the use of incense became an even more integral part of Indian society. Special ceremonies called *yagnas* are held during seasonal transition times. Central to the *yagna* ceremony is the building of special fire pits—called *agni kunds*—of a specific geometric design that acts as a giant censer for aromatic plants. People gather around the fire pits and chant powerful mantras while inhaling the fragrant smoke. This is done as sort of a "public health" ritual that harmonizes the minds and bodies of the community with the Unseen Power (McMahone, 2001).

The Fragrance of Hindu Worship

Hindu rituals are closely connected to the use of fragrant substances. In the temples, as well as on home altars, incense may be burned as sacrifices to the many gods and goddesses of the Hindu beliefs. For example, the god Shiva is honored with the burning of incense every four hours among the religious. Among the most important incense substances in India, and among the Hindu people, is sandalwood. It is used in so many different ways, that its fragrance accompanies every stage of life. Sandalwood is used as a body powder, an oil, a perfume, a wood for "rosary beads" and other carvings, and an incense (Fischer-Rizzi, 1996).

According to ancient Hindu writings, incense and other materials, such as milk and cow products, were used as sacrifices. The Hindu beliefs state that the gods and spirits of ancestors were nourished by the aromas of burnt offerings. The Hindu incense is compounded by several specific substances including frankincense, kungelium (two kinds of rosin), sarsaparilla, *Periploca indica, Curcuma zedoria, Cyperus textilis,* kondo sange-lingam, and the root of the lime tree. Incense is offered freely in the modern Hindu temples. For instance, in the temple of Shiva, incense is offered to the *Lingam*(the phallus) six times during a twenty-four-hour period (Atchley, 1909).

The Holy Fire is an important Hindu ritual, and among the religious it is lighted every morning and evening along with an offering of fragrant incenses. A poem by Kalidasa (fifth century), in Sakuntala, captures the essence of this practice (Fischer-Rizzi, 1996):

> Sacred fires on the consecrated ground,
> nourished by wood, blaze in the hearth around the altar.
> May they, together with the holy sacrifice of fragrance,
> erase my sins and cleanse you!

During the Hindu wedding the Holy Fire is again important, as the ceremony takes place around the Holy Fire. In typical Hindu wedding ceremonies, the couple walks around seven times. In the Malayalam Hindu wedding ceremony, the bride is adorned in flowers, colorful jewelry, and in the sari of a color of her choice. She awaits the groom at her home with a dowry of eight essential items, one of them being a set of sandalwood powder. In the Parsi Hindu wedding ceremony the *aferghaniyu* (a small container that holds smoldering incense sticks) is used to bless the symbolic mango sapling that is planted by the groom and decorated with various other ritualistic offerings.

According to Hindu principles, living a harmonious life also means living with a fulfilling love life. The *Kama Sutra,* a book written in the fourth century AD on the "Instructions in the Art of Love," describes the morning rituals of Hindus of high caste. In the morning they use a fragrant cream on their bodies, a wax mixed with plant juices on their lips, brush their teeth, and wear a flower on their clothing. Fragrances are considered a key element to enhance the love-making experience. The fragrant atmosphere considered to be the optimal for bringing the divine union into fruition according to the *Kama Sutra* is the bedroom that is perfumed by the scent of jasmine garlands, sandalwood incense, and the sweat of lovemaking (Hyams, 2004; Fischer-Rizzi, 1996).

The artful handling of fragrant substances is also considered by the *Kama Sutra* to be one of the essential sixty-four arts that the cultured class needs to learn to do well. Incense was burned in the form of mixtures, powders, *dhoop* (herbs and resins combined into a putty), and incense sticks *(agarbatti)*. Incense in the form of cones or sticks are present throughout the Indian life, on altars, in taxicabs, at markets and vegetable stands, and in homes. Along the sacred Ganges River that originates in the Himalayas are burial sites where large pieces of sandalwood are added to the fire. Sandalwood is thought not only to be an erotically stimulating fragrance, but also to support the journey of the deceased to a more magnificent life (Fischer-Rizzi, 1996).

FOLLOWING THE BUDDHIST PATH TO CHINA

Incense has been present in Asian countries since ancient times. It is normally told that incense came to China first through the spread of Buddhism, and then traveled to other countries from there. This would certainly be true of the use of incense in Buddhism, and how the use of incense spread due to Buddhism. However, it is known that in China aromatic gums, resins, and incense were used since before the introduction of Buddhism into China in religious ancestral worship, with Taoist and Confucian rites. The Chinese ancients mostly were known to use southernwood and mugwort in powdered form to communicate with spiritual beings. The Chinese history of incense use is typical to the rest of the world in that incense use was present in more primitive cultures and rituals long before it was used in the ways we know of today (Bedini, 1994).

Incense use and Buddhism spread together into a number of countries, such as China, Japan, Korea, Burma, Nepal, Tibet, and Sri Lanka. In Japan, incense use was not known in the earlier religion, Shintoism, but later became an important part of the culture. In these Asian and Far Eastern countries, incense use has served religious, secular, and recreational purposes (Bedini, 1994).

The Asian experience of incense spans many uses, including in religious ceremony; in medicine; as an act of consecration; to freshen the air; to cool the body; to scent and perfume the clothing, bedclothes, and hair; as a subject of many literary works and poems; and as a time-keeper. In the oldest known pharmacopoeia, *Hsin-hsiu pents'ao,* from approximately AD 659, the major incense ingredients of early times were listed as aloeswood, frankincense, cloves, patchouli, elemi, and liquidambar. Later, in the Han period, Emperor Wu imported new aromatics (140-87 BC) due to new international relations, and this inspired the invention of the "hill censer," one of the early incense burners. Another form of censer that expanded the use of incense was the *Pei chung hsiang lu,* a censer with gimbals used for perfuming clothes. In the earliest times of censers, they were mostly used to burn artemisia (mugwort and southernwood) and orchids (a fragrant species called lan hui lan, *Cymbidium faberi*). Later, aromatics began to be imported, such as aloeswood, anise, basil, benzoin, ambergris, camphor, cassia, civet, clove, frankincense, jasmine, and storax. One plant, *Perilla ocimoides (P. frutescens),* was favored for use in timekeeping mixtures due to its even and slow burning qualities. Incense sticks, often called joss sticks, were known from early times, and a method of manufacture was employed similar to making noodles. The family that provided the Imperial family with incense in the sixteenth century in China survives today as the company called Nippon Kodo (Bedini, 1994).

The use of incense in sticks, especially in China, is often referred to as "joss sticks." The word "joss" developed after Portuguese traders visited China. They referred to the incense that they saw burning in temples and other places in front of the images of Buddha as "god sticks." Because the Chinese could not easily pronounce their words for "god," which was *deos,* or the Latin word, *deus,* they pronounced it as "joss" instead (Bedini, 1994).

Another development in the Asian use of incense through history was a type of cigarette called the *hangon-kôs* (Herb of Hangon). It was named and fashioned after a type of incense that was used during the Han Dynasty called "spirit-recalling incense" *(fan hun hsiang)*. The popularity of the incense was not so much due to the suggestion of the name being a spirit-summoning incense, but because smoke would cause a photographic image of a dancing girl to appear on the mouthpiece due to smoke while smoking it (Bedini, 1994).

In Japan, a large piece of aloeswood is preserved in the Shosoin, the Imperial Treasury at Nara, measuring approximately 152 cm in length and 122 cm in width at one end, and only 13 cm on the other. It is a piece of high quality aloeswood that is known as the *Ranjatai,* and was a gift from the Chinese court to Emperor Shomu (ruling AD 724-748). Small pieces have been removed from time to time for important and ceremonial occasions (Bedini, 1994).

Prevailing Over the Forces of Evil in Taoism

Gums and resins were used as incense from ancient times in Taoism in China. The purpose of the use of incense in Taoism was multifaceted, and included exorcisms, incantations, and magical rites. Explanations of how it worked varied from its believed ability to make gods indulgent to its effect on scattering evil.

Large standing bronze or cast iron cauldrons are used as stoves or incense burners in the courtyard of Taoist temples. Clusters of incense sticks are inserted into an ash base in the cauldrons and left to smolder. Powdered incense is also used as it is sifted onto ash on flat metal surfaces. A censer that is a long-handled basin *(shou lu)* is also occasionally used in Taoist ritual for burning incense (Bedini, 1994).

One ritual that has not changed since the fifth century, and in which incense use is very important in the Taoist tradition, occurs with its use on the altar. A "furnace master" is chosen, and each liturgy begins with a ceremonial lighting of the long handled incense burner. During the liturgy there is symbolism of the forces of evil trying to steal the incense burner, and the "furnace master" prevailing in keeping it. At the end of the liturgy, there is another ceremonial lighting of the incense burner to represent that the evil forces were defeated (Bedini, 1994).

Buddhist Use and Spread of Incense

A couple of the earliest known materials used as incense in the Chinese tradition were southernwood and mugwort. An "incense water" was also prepared from fragrant incense woods that could be splashed and rubbed on the body to cool it from heat. From the use of early incense materials to communicate with spiritual beings came the ideas that incense brought our prayers on its smoke to the gods, and also that it brought Buddha's mercy to those in prayer. As incense was spread from India along with Buddhism, new types of fragrances and incense materials became known to new areas. This resulted in new customs and beliefs about incense being developed that supplemented the old customs. The result was that incense took on a more prominent role in Buddhist observances and symbolism through its spread to other areas (Bedini, 1994).

Basically, the Chan sect of Buddhism originated from China, and Zen arose when it moved to Japan. A Buddhist sutra called the *Flower Adornment Sutra* (in Sanskrit *Avatamsaka*) talks about the bodhisattva (awakened being) path and how a bodhisattva sees the world. In this, a young man who is wanting to learn the bodhisattva practices and way of life embarks on an epic journey, visiting fifty-three teachers, two of them being incense teachers. As he asks one of the teachers about the bodhisattva path, the Elder named Utpala Flower responds (Tripitaka, 1981, p. 6):

> Good man, I am skilled at discriminating and knowing the myriad of incenses. I also know the methods of blending and mixing all incenses. All incenses means specifically: all burning incenses, all paste incenses, all powdered incenses.
>
> I also know the places from which all the kings of incenses originate. Moreover I am skilled at understanding and knowing the incenses of gods, the incenses of dragons . . . humans and non-humans and so forth—all of those myriad incenses.
>
> Moreover, I am skilled at discriminating and knowing the incenses for curing the myriad illnesses; the incenses for cutting off all evil; the incenses for producing happiness; the incenses for increasing afflictions. The incenses for destroying afflictions; the incenses that cause one to produce pleasure and fixation toward that which is conditioned. The incenses that cause one to produce disgust and the wish to separate from that which is conditioned. The incenses of renouncing all arrogance and self-indulgences; the incenses of bringing forth the resolve to be mindful of all Buddhas; the incenses of certification to and un-

derstanding the different dharma doors; the incense whose use is received by the sages.

From this passage we may see that the use of incense is important for the awakened being in helping other people in many ways. The passage reveals the breadth of knowledge that Buddhism offers about incense. Truly, one could spend more than a lifetime learning the ways of incense.

In Japan, the use of incense began as a secular activity, with at least twenty-four different varieties of wood known before the introduction of Buddhism. The use of incense in Buddhism in Japan began through its introduction as a gift of temple materials by King Song-myong of the Korean kingdom of Paekche to the Japanese Emperor Kinmei. In AD 551 Kinmei became the first Japanese emperor to become interested in Buddhism, and this sparked the spread of Buddhism in Japan. Although earlier missionaries had wandered the country in previous years, Buddhism had not yet taken hold. As more court nobility eventually adopted it as their religion, and Chinese art became popularized, it became firmly established in Japan and many temples were built at and around Nara (Bedini, 1994).

During Japanese Buddhist worship, an inexpensive and common form of incense was burned called *ansokukô,* and more expensive varieties of incense were used by the rich in their temples, such as *ranjatai.* In Japan, as well as other countries, the use of incense in Buddhism was influenced by earlier religious and superstitious beliefs. One example of this is that according to Japanese legend, the burning of incense summons certain demons, called *jikikoki,* or "incense-eating goblins," which are demons that were the souls of men who had in their lifetime sold incense of inferior quality and now sought their food as incense smoke (Bedini, 1994).

In front of temples in Japan, large bronze or iron pots are placed in the courtyard in front of the temple. Each is filled partway with ashes, and incense sticks are inserted into each. As in China, in Japan incense plays an important role in ceremonies surrounding a death. A Buddhist priest will offer: "In my heart's core I respectfully request that the scent of this stick of incense offering from the heart may pervade the regions where the Law prevails and the Messenger of Hades may conduct the soul thither" (Bedini, 1994, p. 46).

Several times a year other memorial rituals are performed for the Buddhist dead, involving the placing of an incense bowl, as well as offerings, a candle, and leaves of the shikimi tree *(Illicium religiosum)* in front of the ancestral tablets (Bedini, 1994).

Incense is also used in the Buddhist ritual of "receiving the fire" *(pul-tatta),* a rite that is performed as the vows for entering the Buddhist priesthood are made. After the head is shaved completely, several cones of incense are placed on the head and burned down to the skin. Painful sores become scars on the heads of monks where the cones burned, and they signify the initiation and are a mark of dedication and holiness (Bedini, 1994).

Japanese homes often have a Shinto altar, and if the family happened to be Buddhist as well they would have a second Buddhist altar. Incense was not traditionally a part of the Shinto altar, which usually was placed above a doorway. However, the Buddhist altar usually included an image of Buddha as well as "soul commemoratives" (remembrances of deceased members of the family), a lamplet, an incense cup, a water vessel, candles, bundles of incense sticks, and sometimes sprays from the shikimi tree. In addition, the incense burner *(koro)* was found on a stand in the main wall of the room, alongside a hanging scroll and a vase of flowers (Bedini, 1994).

In Korea, Buddhism flourished in the seventh and eighth centuries due to the migration of priests from T'ang China. In the fifteenth century it became the state religion and is still present today in its adapted Chinese form. The type of incense known in the temples of Korea is called "longevity incense," which is made from mushrooms that grew on oak trees. It is powdered and placed in trays in a room off the main hall of the temple (Bedini, 1994).

Buddhism and Shamanism in the Himalayas

The Himalayan Mountains are a source of not only awe-inspiring beauty, but according to the Tibetans, of magical and powerful plants that are used for incense among other things. The Himalayan Mountains are thought of as the "seat of the gods," and the clear, thin air seems to carry a spirituality that pervades all of life. Life is conducted in a spiritual way, and incense plays a big role in that from early in the morning (Fischer-Rizzi, 1996).

Incense use that is mostly inspired by Buddhism, and that encompasses all aspects of life like it does in Japan and China, is also found in Tibet, Mongolia, and Manchuria. In Tibet, Buddhism was brought in the seventh century from preachers from India, and what developed there became its own Tibetan form of Buddhism. A number of priests or lamas evolved in Tibet rapidly, and eventually they became the kingship of Tibet, which was ruled by the priesthood in the form of the Dalai Lama. As in China and Japan, incense also became important in many aspects of life, and is offered daily in temples and homes. When incense is not available, juniper sprays are used in its place. In the morning and night outside the entrance of homes, a kiln that sits outside the front door burns juniper, cedar, and sage (Bedini, 1994).

In the Tibetan Buddhist temple, incense is offered as one of the eight essential offerings, part of every rite performed. Incense is also placed around the country, especially in front of crevices on rocky grades, where evil spirits are thought to dwell. On the anniversary of the Buddha's death, incense is burned in Tibet "on every hilltop, and in every temple, home shrine, and lamasery" (Bedini, 1994, p. 51). Imagine what a beautiful sight that is!

Medicinal Incense in Buddhism and Shamanism

Tibetans believe that all illness comes from the insults and illness of the spirit, and that three poisons—greed, hate, and ignorance—are the root cause of all this suffering. Traditional Tibetan medicine treats the mind and the body at the same time, as this is inseparable according to their beliefs. Since incense is clearly a spiritual medicine, it is a key medicine used in treating illness with traditional Tibetan medicine. Specific mixtures for a variety of illness states exist, and certain blends are administered by the Tibetan physicians, while others are more commonplace and useful for keeping the spirit healthy on a daily basis. Some of the ingredients that might be added to a Tibetan medicinal incense mixture might be dark, light, and reddish aloeswood, myrrh, frankincense, nutmeg, raisins, juniper, myrobalan resin (three different types), sal resin, and Chinese larkspur. Other unique aspects of the Tibetan medicinal incense formulations are that they may contain small pieces of feathers, such as from the peacock, owl, or crow, or pulverized precious stones, such as lapis lazuli, ruby, and turquoise. Some of the recipes are very ancient and have been around for centuries (Fischer-Rizzi, 1996).

Tibetan physicians have been trained not only on the more physical aspects of disease, but especially on the spiritual aspects of health and illness, and they are very specific in how the medicinal formulations are applied. One way of applying a medicinal incense is to cover the patient's head with a towel and then have them lean over the towel to inhale, although sometimes this is done without the towel (Fischer-Rizzi, 1996).

Another form of "medicinally used" incense in Tibet is in the area of shamanism. Shamanism and Tantra have a long tradition in Tibet, and have a presence there even today. Incenses—or *dhup* or *duphad-hupa*—are viewed as having a "heavenly," "earthly," or "hellish" scent by the shamans of Nepal. In Katmandu is a street in the Newari district called the street of the *banya*—the caste of the Newari that are specialists in the trade of incense and medicinal plants. On this street of shacks with cans and bags of incense arranged on the floors, many different kinds of people come to buy their incense, including the regular Newari, the shamans and *gubajus* (priests/astrologers/healers of the Newari people in the Katmandu valley), *diobajus* (men of the Newari), as well as Muslims (Muller-Ebeling et al., 2000).

In Nepal, approximately sixty-nine different single incense types that are used to formulate more complex blends. The number one incense plant is considered to be the high altitude juniper *(Juniperus recurva),* also known as incense tree. This tree is sacred to most of the people of the Himalayas, and though the tips are most commonly used, incense braids are also made from the ground-up branches. One of the oldest incenses of mankind, mugwort, is also an important incense plant in Nepal, as it is considered number one among the leafy or herbaceous incense plants. Mugwort is essential in all of the shamanic ceremonies, and may be placed on altars, hung in a bundle in the house, or rubbed on the drum of the shaman. It is considered to be important protection against disease-carrying demons, and used for purification of the "body and house, spirit and yard" (Muller-Ebeling et al., 2000, p. 139).

The Tantric Incense Seal

Tantrism is a sect of Buddhism that was popular in China, and evolved into a more organized form in the seventh century in India. It is based on sacred Buddhist texts called tantra *(ta chiao or shen pien).*

Tantra is known as the "way of the thunderbolt," which is characterized by a strong magical element, mantras ("words of power"), hand
gestures, talismans, and amulets, among other types of charms. It was
officially introduced to China in the eighth century, and possibly because it shares so many aspects with early Taoism, became a popular
sect in China.

Amoghavajra (AD 705-774) was known as the "Master of Tantric
Buddhism," who became the head of a school in China and also developed a new system called Siddham. Siddham involved the replac-
ing of Sanskrit words by Chinese characters, and made it much easier
for the Chinese to understand and adopt aspects of Buddhism. Siddham became much used in both China and Japan and it also formed
the shape of the incense seal.

The incense seal was developed as a feature of one of the tantric rituals which was described in the tantric scriptures, called "The [In-
cense] Seal of AvalokitésvaraBodhisattva." Avalokitésvara is a divinity that is known to have come to earth in many incarnations as a
savior of the faith. In the text, it is described how the incense seal is to
be shaped in the form of a Siddham seal-character and burned. According to the scriptures, "great insight and perfect freedom can be
attained by the utilization and knowledge of secret seals *[mudra]*"
(p. 73). The mold of the seal is detailed to be the combination of the
four letters *ha* (meaning the origin of all being is ungraspably empty),
ra (undefiled purity), *í* (ungraspable freedom), and *ah* (innately un-
born and undying)—to form *hríh*. As the incense seal burns, it then
passes through and encompasses all aspects of existence. The pattern
is known as the "Great Compassion Which Allays Suffering," and
when the incense is burned it manifests the True Principle. When the
incense smoke is consumed it is said to be the "arising and passing of
all things within Emptiness." When a person masters the mantra that
goes with the seal, he or she is said to then enter the undefiled world.
The smoke produces the incense seal pattern that symbolizes the
aspiration for perfect enlightenment (Bedini, 1994).

In Japan, the incense seal of Avalokitésvara is known as the
"*kirikuji* incense burner." This seal symbolizes the Amida Buddha
(Amitabha), or the Buddha of Compassion. Even though the seal has
survived in a number of Japanese temples, it is not really well known,
and not often used by the Japanese Buddhist priesthood (Bedini,
1994).

The Japanese Art of Koh-Do *(The Way of Incense)*

Incense use became popular in Japan first through the influence of Buddhism imported from China. As certain Buddhist rituals required the use of incense, the aristocracy and ruling class that embraced Buddhism early on began to become familiar with its use. This is because Buddhist rituals slowly began to replace the Shinto (Japan's indigenous religion) rituals that were part of state functions and imperial court ceremony. As previously mentioned, among the incense concepts that were imported from China was the phrase "listening to the incense" instead of using the phrase "smelling the incense." This came from the fourteen volume Mahayana sutra of Buddhism, in which everything in Buddha's world—even the words of Buddha himself—is fragrant like incense. In fact, according to the teaching, *incense* and *fragrance* have the same meaning, and so when bodhisattvas were to listen to the words or teachings of Buddha, they were in fact, listening to incense. This expression was first adopted by the Chinese, and then later by the Japanese (Morita, 1992).

By the end of the Muromachi period (1336-1573) in Japan, "listening to the incense" became an established art form called *Koh-do,* and single fragrant woods became more popular than the incense blends themselves. The favored fragrant wood incense in Japan was called *Jinkah,* also called aloeswood (or agarwood), and it was very precious since it had to be imported from special trees that produced it in Southeast Asia. The highest quality *Jinkah* (meaning "sinking wood") actually sank in water because it was laden with fragrant oils (Morita, 1992).

One example of a *Koh-do* game is presented here taken from the *Book of Incense* (Morita, 1992). This game is called The Three Scenic Spots, and is a poetic appreciation game of the three well-known scenic areas in Japan: Matsushima, Amanohashidate, and Itsukushima. Four different types of incenses were used in the game, and each participant listens for them as they are shuffled by the master of ceremonies. If the participant got all four correct, then he is interpreted to see "The Three Scenic Spots." If he got only two correct, then his answer sheet is interpreted as "Evening Mist" because the scenic spots were somewhat obscured by the evening mist. Likewise, only one correct is because the player was obscured by the "Morning Mist," which lingers longer than that of the evening mist. If the one that is correct is interpreted as "Boat," this is said to be because the participant viewed the three spots from boat without having set foot on the land (Morita, 1992).

In the middle of the Edo period (1603-1867) of Japan *Koh-do* was at its peak of popularity. Originating in the aristocracy and shogun class, *Koh-do* spread to the emerging merchant class, and then to some commoners. *Koh-do* even became one of the pastimes that was thought suitable for women to participate in, and some commoner women, including courtesans, mastered it. People scented their robes and hair with incense in order to cover body odor, attract the opposite sex, and to smell of high-quality incense. As it became popular, men were found to scent their robes and hide incense in the sleeves to appear more elegant so they could attract women. *Kyara* was the word for the highest quality *"jin"* incense, and the use of the word spread as a complimentary world, for example, a *kyara* woman was a beautiful woman (Morita, 1992).

As incense use became more popular, it also became more sophisticated and governed by certain rules of etiquette taught by masters through books. Soon this gave rise to the establishment of schools to formally legitimize their teachings, and two of the teachers of that time became the "founders" of two main popular styles of *Koh-do*. One school was headed by Shino Soshin (the Shino School), and it was characterized by its warrior style of discipline to rules and spiritual training, and the other that was headed by Sanjonishi Sanetaka (the Oie School) was characterized as having games of a more courtly and poetic nature. The schools became hierarchical, where the teachers sat at the top of the pyramid, and only the students who reached a certain level of training would be taught the next level of knowledge by the master of the school. Even though textbooks were written about *Koh-do,* due to the secretive nature of the knowledge of the scents and spirituality associated with *Koh-do* they were not included in the texts. Therefore the textbooks were written mostly as a guide for the sequence of steps that were followed during a *Koh-do* ceremony, information on utensils, etc. (Morita, 1992).

In the middle of the nineteenth century, along with Western influence, *Koh-do* and many of the other Japanese arts began to decline. This was due to commercialization and emphasis on ritual and technical skill rather than development of aesthetic elements of the arts. An additional influence that added to the demise of *Koh-do* was the scarcity of materials, as certain incenses became sparse, such as musk and other incense plants. However, a revival of the *Koh-do* ceremonies began in Japan in about 1920, and in 1982, certain masters of *Koh-do* came to the United States to perform *Koh-do* ceremonies. To this date, a small study group remains in Boston, and others are said to be starting around the country (Morita, 1992).

ISRAEL: INCENSE ARISING FROM THE HOLY LAND

In the book of Exodus is the first explanation of the sacredness of incense burning in divine worship, as instructions given to Moses by God. According to this story, the ascending smoke represents "the image of the breath and the name of the Lord" (Fischer-Rizzi, 1996, p. 136).

The Hebrews have long considered incense burning to be sacred, and many people have thought the Hebrew use of incense was where Christianity derived its use and mode of using incense. It is thought that the ritual of incense offering came from the adoption and influence of the Assyrian cults. Indeed, a close resemblance exists between the temples of Babylon and Jerusalem in their features, the daily sacrifice, many of the offerings, libations, and the tables before Yahweh and Marduk respectively. At first the prophetic party did not approve to the adoption of sacrifices and burnt offerings, as they had not yet been ordained by Yahweh. The first censers that were used were handheld, and probably resembled those of the Egyptians with a pan or bowl attached to a long handle (Atchley, 1909).

Those recipes of temple frankincense and sacred oils found in the Kabbalah were used not only to show the connection of the people to God, but to represent God himself. The Kabbalah describes the sacredness and symbolism of the four substances to be used in the Temple, representing the four elements: water, earth, air, and fire. These four incenses are generally thought to be balsam, onycha, galbanum, and frankincense, although there is much difference of opinion as to the exact identity of these "spices" (Fischer-Rizzi, 1996).

In the Torah God spoke to Moses about the use and sacredness of incense after telling him of anointing oil. The incense altar *(Mizbeach HaQetoret),* anointing oil *(Shemen Mish'chat KodeshHaMish'chah),* and incense *(Qetoret)* all represent spiritual levels of the closeness to God. The Hebrew word *Qetoret* represents something that "rises up in circles, and whose aroma wafts and spreads" (Sutton, 2000). In Aramaic, the word means "connection" (Sutton, 2000). God said to Moses:

> Take for yourself spices—balsam, onycha, galbanum, [as well as other specified] spices, and pure frankincense—equal amounts of each. [Grind each spice separately and then] blend [them together as] a *qetoret* compound, the work of a master perfumer, well-blended, free of all impurity, and holy. Pulverize a small portion of [the *qetoret* daily] and place it [on the Golden Altar] before the [Ark of] Testimony in the Communion Tent where I commune with you. It shall have the highest degree of holiness for you *[kodesh kodashim]*. With regard to the *qetoret* you are to make, do not duplicate its formula for your personal use. It must remain separate and set aside for God. If a person makes it to enjoy its fragrance, he shall be cut off [spiritually] from his people. (Exodus 30:34-38; Sutton, 2000)

It is easy to see how incense was also closely associated with the lighting of the menorah. In the original prayer book *(Siddur)* it was also said:

> Aaron must burn the *qetoret* spices on [the Golden Altar] early each morning when he cleans the [Menorah] lamps. He must also burn the *qetoret* when he lights the lamps toward evening. It is a daily *qetoret* offering before God throughout all your generations. (Exodus 30:7-8; Sutton, 2000)

Therefore, in the *Qetoret,* eleven spices make up the mixture—equal parts of balsam, onycha, galbanum, and frankincense—as well as seven others that are identified only in oral tradition. Among these are thought to be myrrh, cassia, spikenard, saffron, cinnamon, costus, and aromatic bark (thought to also be cinnamon). Another concept becomes evident in the Torah of both the incense mixture and the anointing oil: that they are not only holy, but the holiest of the holy *(Kodesh Kodashim)*. They are to be treated separately from ordinary life, as they have the power to elevate everything they touch and infuse it with holy power. Therefore, they are to be treated in a careful way, as they are so powerful as to be dangerous if misused. In the Talmud, Moses also learns of incense by the Angel of Death. It is revealed to him that incense has the power to nullify "any evil decree, even death" (Sutton, 2000).

It was explained that the incense mixture not only has the power to heal, but also the power to bring death. During the plague, Moses asked Aaron to take the fire pan containing the *Qetoret* and to bring it to the community to save them from the wrath of God (being the plague). As he brought it to them and stood between the dead and the living, the plague was stopped. In this mixture, balsam was healing for the body, frankincense signified God's love for his people and how he was able to erase their sins from them, onycha signifies the entire Jewish population, and galbanum alludes to complete sinners (Sutton, 2000).

In the mixture of eleven spices, one spice exists that is not pleasant smelling. According to Rabbi Avraham Sutton (2000), God created a world in which corporeal man could live in a physical environment and have the experience of using his own free will to face temptation and overcome it and reap the ultimate reward. In order to create such an environment for man, first God had to withdraw His Light. To then explain how the incense mixture was composed, he explains that it was made to correspond to the act of God creating the universe (Sutton, 2000).

According to Rabbi Sutton (2000),

> In our prayers every morning, we thus reenact all of history in miniature. The *Qetoret*, especially, placed as it is both at the beginning and the end of the Morning Service, is one of the most important sections of the prayers for effecting redemption. All together, all the different parts of the prayers are the most powerful way to unite the Holy One and His Shechinah, YHVH (26) and Adonai (65). 26 + 65 = 91 = Amen.

The *Qetoret* then not only reveals to us that all is as God planned, but it also has the power to stand up to evil and death and to defeat them, and to transform them into life, and to reveal God's Light (Sutton, 2000).

THE CATHOLIC CHURCH AND CHRISTIANITY

The value and sacredness of incense is prevalent in the Bible. Two of the gifts to baby Jesus were of incense: frankincense and myrrh:

> When they saw the star, they rejoiced exceedingly with great
> joy. And going into the house they saw the child with Mary his
> mother, and they fell down and worshiped him. Then, opening
> their treasures, they offered him gifts, gold and frankincense
> and myrrh. (Matthew 2:10-11, English Standard Version)

The early Church claimed that the use of incense was akin to the worship of idols, and incense itself was "food for demons." Therefore, incense use was banned in the early Church for two hundred years. Personal use of perfume was also thought to be an indulgent luxury that could lead to sensual lust. Thus, as Christianity became popular in the fourth century, the use of perfumes and incense in the Roman Empire declined (Classen et al., 1994; Atchley, 1909).

Although some incense use may have occurred in certain processions, such as funerals, there was basically no incense use in the public worship of the Church until the time of Constantine the Great. The early Church was opposed to following any precedents from the early non-Christian religions, especially the Jewish precedents. Constantine inaugurated The Peace of The Church, and a new era began (Atchley, 1909).

The invasion of Germanic tribes who were unaccustomed to the lavish use of scents regarded the use of scents by the Roman elite as unnecessary niceties, and showed no patience for this kind of primping. However, even though the fall of the Roman Empire led to the loss of many of the olfactory rituals of the Romans, such as scented baths and cloths, the use of scent was so culturally ingrained that some of those beliefs and customs were carried on. Christianity incorporated many of these olfactory practices and beliefs, and incense then was accepted as a symbol of prayer by the sixth century (Classen et al., 1994).

A general change came over the Church in their attitude toward many of the pagan customs. The earliest Christian uses of incense that were documented were at funeral processions, the earliest known to be that of St. Peter of Alexandria in AD 311. Whereas the funerals of the Greeks and Romans (in their pagan days) were characterized by grief and despair because a life had ended, the Church offered a much different teaching. Death now meant that the person was "on to better things," and a reason to rejoice in their last rites. Funerals began to be held during the daytime, instead of during the night, and olive branches and palms were presented as signs of victory in substitution of the cypress, as this was a symbol of mourning. In addition to torches and lights being retained as in a triumphal procession, censers with incense were also carried (Atchley, 1909).

Slowly, with small changes in the Church, more emphasis was invested in the passages of the Old Testament in which God ordained the sacrifice of incense and actually took pleasure in it. By the sixth century, there were documented cases of Christians offering incense as a sacrifice and a propitiation, such as in The Testament of St. Ephraim (Atchley, 1909).

To the Christians, the sacredness of the four incense burning substances—balsam, myrrh, galbanum, and frankincense—symbolized the four parts of prayer: petition, intercession, glorification, and thanks.

According to Father Thomas Scirghi, SJ, Professor of Liturgy at the Graduate Theological Union in Berkeley, California, incense plays a threefold role within worship (see Photo G.6 in the color photo gallery). First, incense provides a visual sign of the prayer of the people rising to the heavens, Father Thomas says, "as found in Psalm 141, 'May your prayers rise like incense.' The sight and smell of the smoke helps to draw the worshipers toward the presence of almighty God." Second, the olfactory sense serves to engage a person in worship as well as to conjure up memories. Father Scirghi recalls his own experience with incense in the liturgy and how the fragrance brings him back to his boyhood and his early memories of attending church with his family in Brooklyn, New York. He can remember the distinct scent of his church and how this experience moved him. Still a third purpose for incense is that of a sign of reverence. Within a liturgical event, the incense is something that indicates it is precious (Father Scirghi, personal communication).

Father Scirghi explains that within the Eucharistic liturgy are three moments in which incense may be used. These moments occur during the three liturgical processions. The liturgy begins with the entrance procession. The thurifer (the person carrying the incense) leads the procession, swinging a thurible (the vessel containing the burning incense). The thurifer is followed by the processional cross, two candle bearers, the Gospel Book, other members of the procession, and finally the presider. This entrance procession, accompanied by the singing of the congregation, serves to gather the people together in praise of God. It is important to note that liturgy should engage all the senses for the purpose of promoting participation in this event. In the procession the worshipers are engaged through sight, sound, and smell. Later they will touch and taste the consecrated bread and wine of the Eucharist (Father Scirghi, personal communication).

The second moment with which incense is used is for the procession of the Gospel Book during the Liturgy of the Word. The Gospel Book is carried from the altar table where it was placed during the entrance procession. While the "Alleluia" is sung, the deacon or priest carries the Book to the ambo (or pulpit), followed by the thurifer. He then announces from which of the four gospels the text is taken. Then he takes the thurible and incenses the Book. He hands the thurible back to the thurifer and proclaims the Gospel (Father Scirghi, personal communication).

The third moment accompanies the procession of the gifts for the preparation of the altar. Here the church prepares for the Liturgy of the Eucharist. The gifts of bread and wine are brought to the table. These will be blessed and become the sacred meal for the believing community. After the altar is set and the gifts are presented to the people, the priest takes the thurible and, swinging it, walks around the table as the smoke fills the sanctuary. Here, it may be noted, that for the early Church the use of incense held a very practical as well as a spiritual purpose. The procession of the gifts includes the collection. Today money is collected in baskets and brought forward with the bread and wine. However, in the early Church, before the use of money, the people would contribute the produce of their livelihood. This included animals and crops. The gathering of all this could create a stench in the sanctuary and throughout the church. The incense helped, then, to mask the odor (Father Scirghi, personal communication).

Having incensed the gifts the priest hands the thurible back to the thurifer. Taking it, the thurifer incenses the priest. After this he descends the steps of the sanctuary, the congregation stands, and he incenses the assembly as well. Here we should take note of the symbolic gesture of incensing. The Church incenses four "objects": the Gospel Book, the bread and wine on the altar, the priest, and the assembly. The fourfold gesture of incensing corresponds with the fourfold presence of Jesus Christ in the liturgy. According to "The Constitution on the Sacred Liturgy," the first document published by the

Second Vatican Council, the Church recognized the presence of Christ in the liturgy specifically in the Word of God, the Eucharistic elements, the minister, and the assembly (Father Scirghi, personal communication).

According to Father Scirghi,

> Sacramental worship provides an opportunity to become aware of the presence of God in our midst. Jesus Christ, the Son of God provides a banquet for his followers. The faithful respond by joining together in a community of prayerful expression. The sight and smell of incense, with its sign and reverence, heighten the awareness of God with His people. (Father Scirghi, personal communication)

Father Scirghi stresses that it is not some kind of magic or illusion that the bread and wine becomes the body and blood of Christ during Communion, but rather it is through our *relationship* with God that we develop faith, and it is this faith that "calls upon the holy spirit to transform ordinary materials of bread and wine into the sacred meal." Therefore, it can be said that if we develop a relationship with the Divine, the Divine may in turn show itself to us in all of our natural surroundings (Father Scirghi, personal communication).

One more clue may lead us to the reason for the use of incense in Christian worship. Author Dudley Hall (1999) elucidated the symbolism of incense and thunder in the book of Revelation as being respectively our prayers and God's answer to our prayers. He explains that the book of Revelation is a symbolic description of Heaven and how we are to mirror our lives to match it. In essence the scripture described a throne with God sitting in it, and when the seals were read, revealing the horrible judgments that were to come upon the earth, seven angels appeared and each were given a trumpet. Another angel who had a golden censer came to the altar and was given a lot of incense to offer that was said to be the prayers of all the saints. This was burned and the smoke went up before God from the angel's censer. When the angel then added to the censer fire from the altar, he threw it down to Earth, and then came thunder, flashes of lightning, and an earthquake. Hall explained,

> Every time we lift our hearts toward God in Jesus' name, an angel of God takes the incense in his hand (our prayers), mixes it

with fire from the altar of God, flings it back to the earth, and it enters the earth's atmosphere as spiritual thunder, lightning, and earthquakes . . . God has chosen to partner with us in transferring heaven into earth. (Hall, 1999, p. 27)

NORTH AMERICA: THE NEW WORLD'S INDIGENOUS INCENSE TRADITIONS

The Native American Sweat Lodge

According to Chief Phil Crazybull, a Native American medicine man and Chief of the Lakota, plants that are used for smoldering are not called incense, but "medicines." They are medicines for the mind, body, and spirit, and they are used every day in the form of smudges (purification) or more occasionally in the various rituals of the Lakota, such as the sweat lodge (*Inipi*ceremony), the Sun Dance, and the Vision Quest, as well as in numerous other tribal rituals (see Photo G.7 in the color photo gallery). He adds,

> Lakota people don't really use "incense." It is my understanding that it (that name) came from books and from people that make the incense and make it a medicine. So they combined all these things together to make it a medicine to help people smell something to keep them connected to the earth, and that is good! It helps people to understand a little bit more about how powerful plants are because a lot of times plants don't emit that much smell, and when you put it in incense form it becomes stronger. And when it becomes stronger people are really able to smell it and it feels good to them, and then if they could relate to it, it becomes a good medicine. And that's what makes incense good to burn in the home, in your cars, or just to burn sometimes so that somebody can smell it, and say "what's that smell" and they will come around. . . . (Chief Crazybull, personal communication, February 2004)

I was lucky enough to be invited to a sweat lodge ceremony for my first time on the West Coast of California. It was being run by a Kurokmedicine man. They told me that if I wanted to learn about the lodge, I needed to experience it directly. So I arrived with a towel and wearing an oversized cotton dress. I entered the lodge, crawling on my hands and knees, and took my place among the circle.

They closed the flap and there was sudden darkness. There we were, a bunch of bodies crammed into a dome, tentlike structure called the sweat lodge, with a pile of heated red-hot lava rocks in a pit at the center of the circle. My heart began to beat with panic, and as singing started, sparks and smoke lit up the lodge, followed by intense heat. More panic. Instantly, I was hoping that the bucket of water in front of me was there to quench my heat, the fire, and my fear, but a splash onto the glowing lava rocks (referred to as *grandfathers*) sent up even more heat—the kind of heat you cannot escape. It took the form of steam and followed the breath into my lungs. With a gasp for air, all I got was fire. *Fire in my lungs!* I thought. More panic. I could only think of how I was going to get out.

So started my first experience in a Native American sweat lodge. My ego being slightly bigger than my fear in that moment, I thought to assess the situation and examine my options—quickly. They told me that this would probably happen, and that if I felt like I wanted to leave I should just pray harder. If that did not work, they told me I should pray even harder and get close to the ground, to Mother Earth. They explained that we were in the womb of Mother Earth, and she would protect me, whatever I went through in the lodge.

So I began to pray. The medicine man, and leader of that sweat lodge ceremony, who is known for his sense of humor as well as good medicine, exclaimed, "Up your nose!" He threw a handful of one of his signature medicines on the glowing hot stones and red sparks lit up the lodge again followed by the intense earthy-sweet smell of powdered wild celery root. I inhaled and thought of the plants. I began to pray to the Creator and to the medicine. An image of the California bay laurel *(Laurus californicus)* trees that hung over the lodge came to me. I remembered the cool, green glow of the moss that grew up their long slender truncks, and I could feel the cool green moss against my burning skin, soothing me. Although to my knowledge no laurel leaves were placed on the rocks, I could feel my lungs cool and open to the remembered scent of the green leaves when crushed.

The scent of laurel leaves is intense to say the least. In fact, it was the basis of one of my favorite tricks to play on hiking buddies. I would begin to earn their trust by crushing and passing a few of the sweet local leaves that we hiked by, while telling them the name of the plants so they could learn their scent. Then I would take a California laurel leaf, crush it, and pass it along. Inevitably, they would whiff the leaf with the same abandon, expecting more sweetness, and be almost knocked to the ground with the cool, camphorous punch of laurel. It's like getting an ice-cream headache through the nose. Holding their noses they would curse me, "Kerry, argh! I am going to get you!"

The laurel plant spirit must have enjoyed our jokes, because today the laurel spirit was with me. It cooled my lungs and opened my breathing. I thought I could endure for a while longer. Then more and more water was poured on the rocks. My skin burned. I tried to sit perfectly still, because each time I moved it was like a fresh blast of fire on the skin. *I am going to burn to death,* I thought. *My skin is actually burning.* The panic started again, and I began to think of getting out. *I can't handle this, I am going to die!* I began praying harder. *Please don't let me die . . . please get me through this experience. I am here to pray. I am here in gratitude, to learn about these ways for my greater understanding of the plants, for purification, healing, and to be closer to the earth. Please don't let me die.* I began to cry in surrender. *Thank you, Creator.*

And that was how my ego was finally set aside during my first *Inipi*lodge. Immediately I felt connected and at ease. *Isn't it strange we have the tendency to look to our higher power only when things get really rough?* I thought afterward, and immediately thought I understood part of the reason for suffering the heat and anxiety.

Native American sweat lodge ceremonies can differ depending on the tribe, leader, or water pourer, of the lodge. Most ceremonies are adaptations of the Lakota (Sioux) sweat lodge ceremony, which has a prescribed tradition in the order and detail of rituals that accompany it. The sweat lodge was gifted to the Lakota by the White Buffalo Calf Woman, who also gave to them the Pipe Ceremony. Traditionally, four herbs accompany the lodge as "incenses" or medicines: cedar, white sage, sweetgrass, and tobacco, which is also used as an offering to the fire and in the ceremonial pipe (*chanupa* or peace pipe). Before entering the lodge, participants, as well as the premises of the lodge, are smudged with white sage or cedar for purification. Traditionally held in a censer that is a simple abalone shell, or as a smudge stick, or other heat-proof receptacle (depending on the tradition), the white sage and/or cedar is burned and the leaves easily give off their plumes of purifying smoke. During the smudge, the smoking sage is often passed from the head down the body to the feet, and then the person turns clockwise around so they can get both sides.

Once smudged, people enter the lodge with women first in the Lakota tradition (actually, according to tradition, only men used to sweat, but today coed lodges are common). Typically, an altar is placed across from the opening of the lodge, which faces west in the Lakota tradition. The medicine man or leader enters the lodge first, then everyone else follows, entering in a clockwise fashion. Once seated, glowing hot rocks (grandfathers) are escorted into the center of the lodge by someone appointed to being a "fire-keeper." As each stone is placed in the pit, it is welcomed with a prayer and cedar and sweetgrass, which fills the lodge with a warm sweet smell. Once the door flap is closed, the incense smoke and steam from water-pouring fill the lodge while the participants pray and sing.

The "incense" plants used in the lodge ceremony are considered medicine, not only for the physical body, but for the spiritual and emotional aspects as well. In fact, it is common for Native Americans to refer to plants used in any ceremonial context as "medicines." They do not see the same division that we tend to see—medicine is for both the spiritual and physical, inseparable from each other.

Indeed, Native American spiritual beliefs have been classified as "animism" because these beliefs include that all parts of nature, including rocks, have spirits. It is the spirit of the plants that do part of the healing.

EUROPE: THE OLD WORLD OF INCENSE

The Celtic Lodge and Surviving European Beliefs

The Celtic people also practiced a sweat lodge that is in many ways similar to the Native American lodge, and in some areas of Europe this tradition is still alive today. Although no written records exist of how the Celtic sweat lodge was built, it has been found in archeological evidence to be two different types of construction: one being a lodge made with wooden poles and animal skins in much the same way the Native American lodge is built, and the other being a lodge constructed in a more permanent way with stones (Fischer-Rizzi, 1996; Andy Baggott, personal communication, November 19, 2004).

The Celts moved into western Europe from 5000 to 4000 BC, and due to their exceptional connection with plants, became enamored with the trees of the forests that then surrounded them. They believed that the plant world was a mystical source of power, and sought spiritual knowledge from plants through the druids and seers who they thought had the ability to directly communicate with the plant world. They saw the life force of plants to be "breathed into them" by elves. These spirits of nature—elves, gnomes, dwarfs, and water nymphs— were seen as helpers that could be accessed for guidance in times of struggle (Fischer-Rizzi, 1996).

The Celts lived among the forest in large, islandlike communities that often included about two hundred people. They did not build churches, but rather received their guidance from priests and priestesses, and they performed their ceremonies in sacred tree groves. In addition, burning incense substances was part of normal life. At the center of every home was an open fireplace, and a house altar that was used for incense mixing and burning. Fragrant resins and woods were borrowed by the Celts from many cultures, including the Etruscans, Romans, and Greeks, and evidence of their importance has been found in archeological finds among grave excavations that showed their belief of these substances accompanying them to the journey beyond (Fischer-Rizzi, 1996).

Beyond the Celtic lodge, other herbal traditions have survived into European culture today. When herbal medicine reemerged in the 1990s, many people in the United States were surprised to learn that certain herbs have been clinically proven to be helpful for many illnesses, and have been a mainstream part of medical therapy in Europe since "Western medicine" began. Herbal medicine was even part of Western culture that the early settlers brought with them to the United States. In the United States this initial presence of herbalism became lost by later movements such as the formation of the American Medical Association (AMA) and later by the movement of incorporating synthetics into pharmacy. In Europe, however, the herbal traditions in pharmacy remained uninterrupted, and are still strong today.

According to Andy Baggott, author of *The Celtic Wheel of Life* and practitioner of Celtic traditions, Celtic beliefs and traditions are very much still alive today. In fact, sweat lodges that are drawn from Celtic beliefs are popular today throughout Europe. Baggott says that many of the Celtic lodges in Europe today bear a resemblance to Native American lodges, and Native Americans have been responsible for coming to Europe and stimulating some of these old beliefs through the teaching of Native American spirituality. Included in the lodge and other Celtic traditions today is the use of incense (Andy Baggott, personal communication, November 19, 2004).

The types of plants used for incense in a Celtic lodge vary, but may include nettle, borage, woodruff, lavender, cedar, and pine. "Coltsfoot is known as British tobacco, and Mullien and lavender are used in this way as well," says Baggott. The Celtic use of incense occurs not only in the sweat lodge, but also in the home. Incense has a long tradition for cleansing the space, as well as the animals and people. In the various Celtic ceremonies and festivals that occur throughout the year, such as for the solstices, equinoxes, and the Fire Festivals (the first days of February, May, August, and November), incense that is used is in harmony with the seasons. For example, rowanberry may be used in autumn for protection; birch, beech, and hazel are related to fertility and used in spring; and yew is used in midwinter (Andy Baggott, personal communication, November 19, 2004).

Other incense-related herbal traditions that have survived into modern European use include the "herbal bouquet" that is part of southern German tradition. This is a bouquet that is gathered and braided together on The Day of Assumption (August 15) made of special herbs whose use date back to Celtic times. The bouquet is consecrated by a priest in church, and then it is placed on the house altar next to a crucifix. A few pieces are picked off and burned, usually with frankincense. The herbs are thought to have healing powers, and the bouquet is burned throughout the year and also on the Day of the Three Kings (January 6) (Fischer-Rizzi, 1996).

FROM THE HIGH ANDES TO DEEP IN THE RAINFOREST: INCENSE USE IN SOUTH AMERICA

Rainforest Shamanism and Other Native Cultures

In Mexico, Central America, and South America the ancient cultures of the Aztec, Maya, and Inca flourished, and many say they were at the peak of their civilizations between the third and sixteenth centuries. Of course, many people know that the Spanish conquistadors were responsible for massive sickness and deaths among these cultures, but what many people do not know is that these cultures are still alive today. These cultures were very sophisticated with their knowledge of medicine and were recorded by botanists of the time to know thousands of plants for medicinal use. The Maya also had the "Book of the Community," the *Popol Vuh,* which detailed the use of plant substances and aromas, such as one called copal (Fischer-Rizzi, 1996).

Among the most widespread and important of the incense substances in Mexico and Central and South America is copal. Copal is one word that refers to a number of plant resins that are used in a similar way in different areas throughout this region. The generic use of the word *copal* is confusing, as it refers to the resins of many species. However, at the same time it generalizes and simplifies the way copal is used through Latin America. Native people of these regions use copal as food for the gods, and still today it also has a strong association with maize, which is considered food for humans. Depending on the species of tree the copal is from it may also be used in other ways, such as for chewing, gluing, as a pigment binder and a varnish, and for purifying meat. Beyond the use by the indigenous people in many of these areas, copal is burned in Catholic churches in a similar way to frankincense.

Since the use of copal spans such a large area, and copal is of several general types and from different trees, its uses are very diverse and dependent on these factors. In the southern Huasteca region, Nahuatl speakers use copal incense for divination. Depending on the location, the shaman may interpret the patterns of smoke coming from the copal, or the shaman might pick up fourteen grains of corn and hold them in the incense smoke. After chanting and asking the spirits to guide him, he will cast the grains onto a cloth and interpret their pattern where they fall. In Mitla, Oaxaca, the Zapotecs may burn copal in water to diagnose the cause of *susto,* or fright, one of the main causes of disease in Latin American folk medicine (Stross, 1997)

In her book, *The Energy Prescription,* Connie Grauds talks about *susto* and how it can be cured through ritual of singing sacred healing songs (called *icaros*) and blowing tobacco smoke or copal over the head of someone with *susto.* In the book Grauds gives an example of a baby who had *susto,* and how its healing involved healing of other members of its family who were unknowingly transmitting their *susto* to the baby (Grauds, personal communication, May 5, 2005).

The shamans representing different tribes in the rain forest regions of Latin America and South America have also been known to enter trance states during the inhalation of incense smoke. Some forms of these incenses are well known today to possess psychoactive and hallucinogenic properties, whereas others are more mild incenses that are not considered to have these properties, such as copal (Stross, 1997).

The rituals and customs for which copal is used are numerous, and indeed the native peoples of the Mesoamerican regions use incense in many ritual occasions. Copal may be used to cense and purify specific sacred objects, such as saint images, clothes, altars, crosses, and community banners. This custom—although it has found its way into many of the adapted forms of Catholicism—was also present before and during the time the Spanish conquistadors arrived (Stross, 1997).

The Ayamara Andean People

The Ayamara live in the high Andes of South America. According to Rufino Paxi (Paxi, Personal Communication, May 22, 2004), a traditional healer/priest *(Amauta),* incense is used as offerings to the cosmos—"to the sky above and to the universe." Rufino says that spirits are present in the universe, nature, animals, all the plants, and even in money, and that incense is a healthy food for these spirits. He is careful to point out that not all incenses are good for indoor use because of safety issues. In the Andes, they use some incenses on the mountaintops that are appropriate only for outdoors, and are good for communicating with ancestors. However, others, such as copal, are suitable for indoor use and even medicines. Incense plays an integral part of Ayamara ceremonies, and for communication with the ancestral world.

Candomble and African-Rooted Religions

The Atlantic slave trade strongly influenced the population and culture of South America, notably Bahia, Brazil. Despite the oppressive and dehumanizing influences of slavery, the middle passage, and the oppressive social structure in the areas to which they were brought, Africans were able to bring the roots of their languages, religions, and spiritual practices with them to influence the Americas. Not only did the religious and ethnomedical practices of Africans survive, but they expanded their geographical ranges and influenced local cultures. The Haitian vodun, also known as "voodoo," "hoodoo," "juju," "root work," or "conjure," spread from its introduction in New Orleans to areas of the northeastern and southeastern United States. Cuban Santeria, which stems from Yoruba beliefs, moved to Florida, then on to New York, California, Spain, and Venezuela. Umbanda, an Afro-Brazilian religion, has been estimated to reach the amount of thirty million, mostly white, middle-class followers. Candomble is another of the Afro-Brazilian religions that mostly is present in areas of eastern and southern Brazil (Voeks, 1997).

Due to the large geographic spread and the evolution and incorporation of local beliefs into these "neo-African" religions, they are described as sharing more differences than similarities. Robert Voeks (1997), author of *Sacred Leaves of Candomble,* describes them as being practical and hedonistic, and mostly dealing with the resolution of earthly problems in the here and now.

In the religion of Candomble, as in several other of the neo-African religions, the followers recognize a supreme creator god, but other gods are worshiped as well. Since the supreme creator, *Olórun*is thought to be unapproachable and distant to humans, the followers of Candomble are more focused on the worship of other gods, called *Orixás,* many of which are closely associated with natural phenomena and processes. Incense is used in the worship of the *Orixás,* in the Candomble ethnomedicine, and in the ceremonies in which the *Orixás* inhabit in a possession trance some of the members of a particular Candomble community, called a *terreiro.* Among these incenses are copal and the leaves of *dendê,* African oil palm or *Elaeis guineensis,* whose leaves are burned in order to chase away bad spirits (Voeks, 1997).

AFRICA: THE ORIGIN OF MAN AND INCENSE?

This sampling of incense rituals and uses throughout the world ends in Africa, quite possibly the real origin of incense use. Most people discuss the origins of incense as coming from Arabia originally and spreading through Asian and European cultures. However, as we look closer at the uses of "incense" in the indigenous religions of

South and North America, we see that incense has quite possibly been in use long before its spread from Arabia. Indeed, as Africa represents the roots of all mankind, as well as being home to the Arabian world (from Morrocco to the eastern part of Africa), it is most likely the birthplace of our use of incense. It is known that in pre-Islamic times sandalwood was used in northern Africa, as well as in the Middle East and the Mediterranean, to ward off evil spirits.

Today, African indigenous religions and spiritual belief systems exist in Africa along with the other major world religions. Muslim and Christian influences have undoubtedly influenced the use of incense in Africa today. Africa now also supplies many of the aromatic resins to the rest of the world, such as frankincense.

As in Sudan at the end of a meal, I will end this chapter by lighting my incense burner containing sandalwood, and let it fill the room with its relaxing delicate fragrance.

Chapter 4

Types of Raw Incense

Real incense is the scent that comes from burning or smoldering parts of plants. Therefore, at its most basic level, incense comes from either plant leaves, bark, resin, or other plant parts. To gain a better understanding of the spiritual or beneficial qualities of incense, it is best that people get to know the source plant of the incense—the raw incense—before it is made into cones, sticks, or other incense forms. This chapter is intended to give a description of the history and background as well as the botanical identification, origins, and chemical components of the major incense types on the market. The incense plants mentioned here are representative of many areas of the world, and are intended to give you a sense of the worldwide phenomena of the most spiritual use of plants that incense represents.

AGARWOOD (ALOESWOOD/JINKOH/EAGLEWOOD): PROMOTING THE SOUL'S DEVELOPMENT TO ITS HIGHEST LEVELS

Scientific names: *Aquilaria* spp. (esp. *A. malaccensis, A. agallocha, A.hirta, and A.beccariana*) and sometimes *Gonystylus bancanus* are the trees infected with fungus (e.g., *Aspergillus* sp. and *Fusarium* sp.).

Common names: Aloeswood, *jinkoh,* eaglewood, *gaharu* (Indonesia), *Chim-Hyang* (Korean), *Chen-Xiang* (Chinese).

Plant family: Thymelaeaceae.

Origin: Korea, Assam, Bhutan, Cambodia, Vietnam, Singapore, Indonesia, Northern India, China, Papua New Guinea.

See Photos G.8 and G.9 in the color photo gallery.

The Incense Bible
© 2007 by The Haworth Press, Inc. All rights reserved.
doi:10.1300/5820_04

Agarwood is a strange and much sought after incense that is produced as a defense mechanism in the wood of a tree that has been harmed or infected by a fungus. Excess resin production results in response to the fungal attack, and the incense is a special combination of the fungus and the defense resin, which produces a specific range of scents. Therefore, the raw incense product looks like slices of wood that have dark striations due to the resin and fungal association. Usually the darker the piece of agarwood, the higher the quality, indicating more resin production. However, there has been some adulteration in quality in Asia by treatment of the wood with dyes to produce a dark color, and glues or other materials to make the wood heavier. In Japan it acquired the name *jinkoh,* meaning "sinking wood," because of its resin-laden quality that causes the wood to sink. Only the better quality *jinkoh,* or agarwood, sinks when immersed in water (Robert Blanchette, personal communication, February 2004; Venkataramanan et al., 1985).

The methods used to differentiate the different types of *jinkoh* traded on the market are complicated, and still being determined. The wood part of agarwood is characterized by the presence of phloem tissues differentiated in the xylem tissue, in addition to the usual secondary phloem derived from cambium. In higher quality samples and types of agarwood, the resin-producing cells were found extending from the phloem into medullary rays and then onto xylem tissues, because the resin content increased. However, in lower quality samples the resin-producing cells were found only in the phloem tissues in xylem (Shimada and Kiyosawa, 1984). Scientists in Japan and other areas of agarwood trade have published a number of studies on the differences between different types of agarwood traded on the market, mostly using essential oil chemistry research and thin layer chromatography (Yamagata and Yoneda, 1986a,b; Yoneda et al., 1986).

Substantial evidence indicates that the numbers of *Aquilaria* trees are decreasing rapidly in recent years. Although *Aquilaria malaccensis* (the main source of the resin) has been listed by the Convention on International Trade in Endangered Species to be monitored for international trade, there is concern that not enough controls are being implemented. One recent report indicated that because the main source of agarwood, which used to be Sumatra and Kalimantan, has recently switched to eastern Indonesia (Maluku and Irian Jaya), and because traditional harvesting practices by locals are being replaced by more intensive harvesting practices by nonlocals, the trade is not sustainable. In addition, reports exist that much of the higher value, high-grade material is thought to be traded illegally and by personal transaction. As a remedy, some recent attempts have been made at making plantations of agarwood with artificially infected trees to produce resin (Robert Blanchette, personal communication, February 2004; Soehartono and Newton, 2002).

Dr. Robert Blanchette, professor in the Department of Plant Pathology, University of Minnesota, has been working on a project in Southeast Asia and has found a way to commercially produce agarwood trees in plantations. It is the hopes of this project to not only provide a sustainable wholesale source of agarwood, but to also help rural peoples of this part of the world make a living in harvesting this endangered tree now in cultivation (Robert Blanchette, personal communication, February 2004). This project recently announced that their first sustainably produced, plantation-grown agarwood is now available for sale on a retail Web site (see Appendix A).

Agarwood has different common names in different countries, and different identified quality grades tend to be country specific and not necessarily easy to distinguish by the amateur because they are based on more qualitative characteristics. In general, agarwood is priced according to the strength of the aroma, size of the pieces of wood, and the degree of blackness (Langenheim, 2004). Six main varieties or qualities of agarwood exist on the market in Japan, each named after traditional groups in Japanese society. Although all are considered high quality, *Kyara* is usually considered the best:

- *Kyara* is considered the most valuable type of agarwood. The heaviest variety and the most laden with fragrance, *Kyara* has been described as "a dignified, gentle fragrance with a slightly bitter tone." It is the aristocrat (Fischer-Rizzi, 1996, p. 205; Morita, 1992).
- *Rakoku* has been described as "a tangy, biting fragrance that reminds one of sandalwood." It is the warrior (Fischer-Rizzi, 1996, p. 205; Morita, 1992).
- *Manaka* has been described as "a bright, tempting fragrance; changeable" (Fischer-Rizzi, 1996, p. 205; Morita, 1992).
- *Manaban* is "usually sweet, but sometimes rough and boorish." The presence of a sticky, oily residue left on the plate is a sign of *Manaban*. It is the peasant (Fischer-Rizzi, 1996, p. 206; Morita, 1992).

- *Sumotara* has "a sour fragrance at the beginning and the end. It is easily mistaken for Kyara . . . sometimes (with an) offensive and uncouth background." This is the servant who is pretending to be the aristocrat (Fischer-Rizzi, 1996, p. 206; Morita, 1992).
- *Sasora* has "a cool and somewhat sour fragrance . . . sometimes it is light and gentle, almost unnoticeable." It can be mistaken for *Kyara,* especially when it is first lit. It is the monk (Fischer-Rizzi, 1996, p. 206; Morita, 1992).

In Indonesia agarwood is traded under the common name of *gaharu.* Although the Indonesian government recognizes only two grades of *gaharu* for export figures, the trade intraregionally is divided into six to eight classes of product, depending on intuitive determination of resin content. Ranked generally in higher to lower grades, they are: Super A, Super B or AB, Super C or BC, *tanggung, teri kacang padat, teri timbul, teri layang,* and *kemedangan.*

Description of Plant

The *Aquilaria* tree is commonly said to look like an eagle with outstretched wings in the way the branches are formed (Fischer-Rizzi, 1996). *Aquilaria* trees are fast growing, and many species are able to make the resin. The most resinous and high quality pieces of agarwood are those trees that have long ago fallen, were buried by leaves and organic matter, and began to decay and produce resin. When this occurs, the woody parts of the plant are mostly decayed, and the resinous pieces remain intact—almost petrified. Some of these pieces have been unearthed after hundreds of years to become the most expensive of the incenses.

Historical and Current Usage

The resinous wood of agarwood has been referred to in the Bible, and is often mistaken as aloe. The word for incense in Sanskrit is *agarbhatti,* of which agar forms the basis of the word, referring to agarwood.

Asia

Jinkoh is the most important of the incenses to Japan. *Jinkoh,* as agarwood is called in Japan, is considered to be the finest scent of the incenses, and is used not only in Buddhist rituals and meditation, but also for the unique Japanese "ceremony" or game called *Koh-do*. The legend of how agarwood came to Japan is that a piece of the wood washed up on the shore of the island of Awaji during the seventeenth century AD, and this wood was presented to the emperor due to its exquisite fragrance when burned. Some versions of the legend say the emperor was already familiar with the wood, and others say he became so enraptured by the fragrance that he started importing it in large quantities (Fischer-Rizzi, 1996).

As discussed in previous chapters, due to the longstanding relationship of Buddhism to incense in China, in Japan they refer to the act of smelling or appreciating incense to "listening to the incense." According to some Buddhists, one can learn all of the teachings of Buddha by just "listening" to the incense. Listening to the incense became such a cherished activity in Japan that the Japanese art of *Koh-do* was developed. This is an intricate ceremony that is comprised of a number of "games" in which the participants "listen" to the incense, and then guess which incenses are present in blends, and write poems describing the identity of incense in a blend.

Agarwood has also long been used in traditional Chinese medicine as a sedative. Active components in agarwood thought to be responsible for this sedative effect are *jinkoh*-eremol and agarospirol. When tested in mice, a benzene extract of agarwood showed a prolonged effect on the sleeping time (hexobarbital-induced) and hypothermic effects, as well as exhibiting other sedative-like qualities. The *jinkoh*-eremol and agarospirol have also been found to be neuroleptic, or useful for treating chronic psychosis (Okugawa et al., 1996).

Although it has a high rate of adulteration, agarwood is used in Nepal by shamans. In the mundum shamanic path, agarwood is invoked at the beginning of every shamanic session by a mantra. Its aroma also brings the shaman back from a deep trance. It is thought to be related to the substance of pleasure and to be directly related to the shamanic Hindu deity Garuda, who has been said to have discovered its medicinal qualities (Muller-Ebeling et al., 2000).

In 1993, Japanese scientists studied the physiological effects of *jinkoh* and found it to be strongly sedative and able to extend sleep periods. In addition, in 1997 aqueous extracts of *jinkoh* were found to be inhibitory to the hypersensitivity reaction by inhibiting the release of histamine from mast cells. Even though it is very popular in Japan, no commercial *jinkoh* is grown there; it is entirely imported from China and other areas of Southeast Asia (Kim et al., 1997; Okugawa et al., 1993).

The Arab World

As in Japan, agarwood has similar associations of being the most cherished of incenses in the Arab world, and is thought to promote the soul's development to its highest levels. In this part of the world it is referred to as *ud* (also Oud), and it is used in Islamic festivities, such as the twenty-seventh day of Ramadan (the celebratory feast for the birth of the prophet and the conclusion of fasting). In Morocco, *ud* is burned on the day of a child's naming, and the Sufi burn the oil or wood during ritual activities of the initiation of the soul into the greater mysteries of life (Fischer-Rizzi, 1996).

Agarwood is said to be

> hot and dry in the third degree. It opens obstructions, breaks winds, disperses excess moisture, strengthens the intestines, invigorates and gladdens the heart, and is beneficial for the brain. It strengthens the senses, restricts the belly, and is beneficial for incontinence originating from cold of the bladder (Johnson, 1998).

It is used as a fumigant alone, or mixed with other substances. When it is mixed with camphor it has medicinal significance as a fumigant, as it can purify the essence of the air. The essence of the air is important because it is believed to be essential for good health (Kim et al., 1997; Johnson, 1998).

Israel

The Bible mentions the agarwood tree (or aloeswood) and incense quite often, but it is often confused in translation with "aloe." Since the agarwood trees grow in northern India, it has been known since antiquity by Christian and Jewish religions. Kings held this fragrant substance so precious that they would scent their clothes, rooms, and beards with it (Fischer-Rizzi, 1996).

Known Chemical Constituents

Sesquiterpenes are known to be responsible for part of the character-istic scent of agarwood. Three types of agarwood with different chemi-cal variation have been identified in the literature. The first, "type A," from *Aquillaria agallocha,* was characterized more than twenty years ago by Indian chemists and known to have two major sesquiterpenes, agarol and agarospirol, along with (-)-selianic furanoids. The second, "type B," from an uncertain species of *Aquillaria* (possibly *A. malac-censis*), contains eight major sesquiterpenes, jinkohol, agarospirol, kusunol, jinkoh-eremol, jinkohol II, ∝-agarofuan, (-)-10-epi-γ-eudes-mol, and ozo-agarospirol. Both are typical in the marketplace. A third, more expensive, kind of *jinkoh* wood, called *Kanankoh,* has been chemically characterized to include (+)-karanone, (+)-dihydrokara-non, and oxo-agarospirol. Agarwood oil is also known to have valen-cane-, eremophilane-, and vetispirane-derivatives. *Kanankoh* was found to have three chromone compounds that other *Jinkoh* did not contain: 2-[2-(4'-methoxyphenyl)ethyl]chromome, 6-methoxy-2-[2-(4'-metho-xyphenyl)ethyl]chromone, and 2-(2-phenylethyl)chromone (Yoneda et al., 1984; Ishihara, Tsuneya, Shiga et al., 1991; Ishihara, Tsuneya, and Uneyama, 1991; Ishihara et al., 1992, 1993; Naef et al., 1992, 1995; Yamagata and Yoneda, 1987).

Various thin-layer chromatography techniques (i.e., discriminate and differential analysis) and gas chromatography-mass spectrome-try (GC-MS) are used to characterize the quality differences between different types of agarwood traded on the market. For example, in Chinese agarwood *(Aquilaria sinensis)* the compounds jinkohol and jinkohol II could not be detected, and no anatomical differences were found between *Aquilaria sinensis, A. agallocha,* and *A. malacensis* (Yoneda et al., 1984; Yoneda, Yamagata, Sugimoto, et al., 1986; Yoneda, Yamagata, and Mizuno, 1986).

Agarwood also contains a number of chromone compounds, along with the following, isolated from the ether extract of agarwood: 6-methoxy-2-(2-(3-methoxy-4-hydroxyphenyl)ethyl)chromone, 6,8-dihydroxy-2-(2-phenylethyl)chromone, 6-hydroxy-2-(2-(4 hydrox-yphenyl)ethyl)chromone, 6-hydroxy-2-(2-(2-hydroxyphenyl)eth-yl)chromone, 7-hydroxy-2-(2-phenylethyl)chromone, 2-(2-phenyl-ethyl)chromone (otherwise known as flidersiachromone), and 6-

hydroxy-7-methoxy-2-(2-phenyl-ethyl)chromone (Konishi et al., 2002).

BALSAM OF PERU/BALSAM OF TOLU:
TWO SOOTHING INCENSES WITH SIMILAR NAMES

Scientific names: *Myroxylon balsamum* (L.) Harms var. pereirae (syn. *M. pereirae*)/*Myroxylon balsamum* (L.) Harms var. balsamum (syn. *M. toluifera*).

Common names: Balsam of Peru or Peru balsam/balsam of Tolu or Tolu balsam; *chuchupate* (Mexico and United States).

Plant family: Fabaceae.

Origin: Northern part of South America; however, balsam of Peru's range extends up into Central America, whereas balsam of Tolu is found primarily in Colombia, with the best quality trees found along the Magdalena River near the city of Santiago de Tolu.

See Photo G.10 in the color photo gallery.

Balsam of Peru is a dark brown resin with a vanilla and cocoa flavor. Balsam of Tolu is a soft resin that is more liquid than the Peru balsam and it has a fragrance that is said to contain the aroma of vanilla, cinnamon, and freshly mowed grass (due to the coumarin content). The balsam of Tolu is valued for its hyacinth-like scents that blend well with floral and oriental compounds (Konishi et al., 2002). Care should be taken when purchasing balsam of Peru, as adulterants are on the market that contain synthetic esters, and these should not be used for incense burning purposes (Fischer-Rizzi, 1996).

The chemical composition of balsam of Peru can vary depending on the origin, as reported by thin-layer chromatography and GC-MS studies (Monard and Grenier, 1969). In central and northern Mexico and the southwestern United States, balsam of Peru may be sold as *chuchupate,* as an alternative for *Ligusticum porteri* (Linares and Bye, 1987).

Description of Plant

Balsam of Peru and balsam of Tolu are different varieties of the same tree species. The balsam of Peru tree grows to be sixty to sixty-five feet, whereas Tolu grows to about only forty feet. Balsam of Peru resin is stimulated in the tree for collecting by knocking on the tree. The bark is generally peeled from the tree and then rags are used to soak up the sap, which is later boiled to release the resin. The Tolu resin is collected by cutting V-shaped incisions in the trunk of the tree, with a calabash container placed at the bottom of the V in order to collect the resin (Fischer-Rizzi, 1996).

Historical and Current Usage

Both resins are used as incenses and traditional medicines, as well as fragrances. In the sixteenth century Popes Pius IV and V gave official permission to substitute balsam of Peru for the much harder to find Mecca balsam for ceremonial incense use, as well as for the sacred anointing oils. In folklore, balsam of Peru is thought to attract wealth and happiness, promote creativity and dream work, and to protect against emotional excess. In addition to ceremonial and fragrant incense purposes, balsam of Peru has been used medicinally in the form of the resin, and also the incense has been used medicinally, especially by the Maya. It is mostly associated with protection and healing of the kidney and bladder, for regulating irregular menstruation, and for soothing colds (Fischer-Rizzi, 1996). It may be mixed with other substances and used to relieve aches and pains, including muscular aches and arthritis (Quezada, 2003). Balsam of Peru is still used locally for asthma, catarrh, rheumatism, diarrhea, and hemorrhoidal pain. Peru balsam has been studied for its use in wound healing, and has been found to lessen scarring. Balsam of Peru is the variety of *Myroxylon* that is most valued medicinally (Langenheim, 2004; Mabberley, 1997).

Balsam of Tolu is enjoyed as an incense substance for its comforting, calming, and harmonizing quality, and it is thought to be able to heal and comfort emotional and "inner" wounds. Balsam of Tolu was once used for embalming. Tolu has also a long medicinal history, not only as a traditional medicine, but it has been used in Europe (officially listed in the 1882 Pharmacopoeia) as a remedy for coughs and colds since it is an antiseptic and has the ability to dry up mucus. Traditionally, Tolu balsam has been used by the Colombians to treat wounds and to stop bleeding. Balsam of Tolu is still used commercially in ointments and is also a flavoring agent (e.g., for cough syrup), as well as a topical antiseptic agent. The Swiss and British pharmacopoeias still list Tolu balsam for use as a simple tincture. Balsam of Tolu and balsam of Peru also are used as a cigarette additive in some countries (Quezada, 2003; Akisue, 1969). Because balsam of Peru is used in a number of fragrance blends (perfumes), it is one of the main fragrances for which allergenic patch testing is performed when people are suspected to have fragrance allergies. In one study of 2,660 patients, 144, or 5.4 percent, were positive for producing allergic reactions to balsam of Peru (Wohrl et al., 2001).

Known Chemical Constituents

Balsam of Peru is primarily made up of peruresino-tannol and benzoic and cinnamic acids and their esters. It also contains cinnamyl cinnamate (or styracin), benzyl cinnamate (or cinamein), and benzyl benzoate (Langenheim, 2004). A number of isoflavonoids have been characterized from balsam of Peru, including calycosin, 2'-hydroxy-7,3',4'-trimethoxyisoflavanone, and 2'-hydroxy-7,3',4'-trimethoxyisoflavone (Maranduba et al., 1979).

Balsam of Tolu is more fluid than Peru balsam because it has greater quantities of phellandrene and alcohols, such as guaiacol and creosol (Langenheim, 2004). In balsam of Tolu, two epimeric 1(5),6-guaiadienes have been characterized, as well as triterpenoids (Friedel and Matusch, 1987; Wahlberg et al., 1971; Wahlberg and Enzell, 1971). Part of the characteristic fragrance of both resins is due to the coumarins (Akisue, 1972a,b).

BENZOIN: A SWEET, FAST-BURNING FRAGRANCE

Scientific names: Benzoin Sumatra—*Styrax benzoin* Dryander (also *S. paralleloneurus*); Benzoin Siam—*Styrax tonkinensis* (Pierre) Craib ex Hartwich (not to be confused with the incense "Storax" from *Styrax officinalis*).

Common names: Kemenyan, kemanyan (Malaysian); kamyan, kumyan (Thai); kam nhan, nyan, yan (Lao); gum benjamin, gum benzoin; sometimes also misleadingly called frankincense (in Indonesia).

Plant family: Stryacaceae.

Origin: Indigenous to Sumatra; other species from tropical Asia are also used for the manufacture of the incense (Quezada, 2003).

May be harvested from India, Sumatra, Java, Cambodia, Laos, and Thailand. Singapore is the major international trading center for benzoin (Kashio and Johnson, 2001; Fischer-Rizzi, 1996).

See Photo G.11 in the color photo gallery.

Benzoin is a resin that is obtained from wounding the bark of trees, and it has a soft, sweet fragrance that resembles vanilla. The resin is extracted from trees by wounding the cambium of the tree repeatedly. The resin is produced as yellowish white tears, with the whitest being of higher quality. The benzoin from Siam (Thailand) is sweeter than that of Sumatra, and it is the more precious and expensive of the two. The "benzoin" is actually a purified portion of the "resinoid"—commonly called benzoin—that is obtained through an extraction (usually alcohol) process (approximately 3 kg resinoid produces 1 kg benzoin). For incense burning, the resinoid is usually used because it is more solid. Benzoic acid (a preservative for foods, drinks, fats, and pharmaceuticals) is now a synthetic product that once was extracted from Sumatra benzoin.

Siam benzoin is generally exported in a raw form just as it is collected, after cleaning and grading. It is usually an orangish/cream color, and milky white when broken. It may also vary to a dark brown color with a glassy appearance. Sumatra benzoin is similar in appearance to the Siam benzoin, but it usually has darker, dirtier looking parts, consisting of a lower grade material. A semiprocessed, low-grade form of block benzoin with pieces of damar embedded in it is commonly found in trade, especially between Indonesia and Singapore (Kashio and Johnson, 2001). Since benzoin gum can be obtained from several different *Styrax* species, analytical methods have been developed to determine the source species from the resin alone (Pastorova et al., 1997).

In general, the higher grades of benzoin are used for creating fragrances, which also translates into more Siam benzoin being used for this purpose. Some perfumers believe that Sumatra benzoin is adulterated as Siam benzoin by adding vanilla to it. However, Sumatra benzoin should not be seen as a lower quality type of benzoin, because it has its own merits and characteristics that are sometimes sought after (Kashio and Johnson, 2001).

Description of Plant

Benzoin is produced from several species from the genus *Styrax* (Styracaceae). The three areas of distribution of the resin are southeastern Asia, southeastern North America to South America, and the Mediterranean (one species). Siam benzoin is derived from *S. tonkinensis,* whereas Sumatra benzoin comes from two species—*S. benzoin* and *S. paralleloneurum.* Other species are known to be tapped for local use in certain areas of Asia, but they are not known to enter trade (Kashio and Johnson, 2001).

The *Styrax* species that benzoin is derived from grows in the form of tall trees. *Styraxtonkinensis* is a deciduous tree that can reach up to twenty-five meters (about eighty-two feet), with smooth, gray bark when young, and brown rough bark as it reaches maturity, with a thirty-centimeter diameter trunk. The trees produce flowers and fruits, and due to *S. tonkinensis's* pioneering nature, its natural range has been expanded to areas of human disturbance of the forest and areas of shifting cultivation (Kashio and Johnson, 2001).

Historical and Current Usage

Benzoin has a long history of use in several cultures, not only as a ceremonial incense burning substance, but also for its medicinal use and as a fragrance. Along with sandalwood it makes one of the most popular mixtures for incense burning in Asia. It's especially noted for its long history of traditional medicine use for coughs and as an antiseptic. It is also used as a flavoring agent in cigarettes (Quezada, 2003). Although it was originally from Southeast Asia (Sumatra, Thailand, and Laos), it was transported to Egypt by Indian merchants, and then later it was included along the frankincense route (Fischer-Rizzi, 1996).

Since Benzoin burns quickly, it is usually preferred to be burned in mixtures, as it does not have time to develop its sweet fragrance otherwise. If it is desired to be experienced alone, it is recommended that benzoin be burned on aluminum foil over charcoal. Benzoin is thought to stimulate and inspire creativity, but it is also soothing and sensuous, appropriate for creating a nurturing and sensual mood. Benzoin is one of the primary sweet and heavily erotic fragrances that is almost always used in incense mixtures in Eastern cultures due to its pleasing and protecting qualities. These mixtures of fragrances are used in protection against the evil eye, and for expelling negative energies and attracting the positive energies. The essential oil of *S. tonkinensis* has been found to exhibit antifungal activity (to both *Aspergillus niger* and *A. flavus*), and the benzoic acid esters are hemolytic (Fischer-Rizzi, 1996; Sangat-Roemantyo, 1990).

Benzoin is traded internationally for the manufacture of flavor and fragrances and for pharmaceutical use. The fragrance industry uses benzoin for both the fragrance it imparts as well as its function as a fixative for decreasing the volatilization of middle and top notes. The food industry uses benzoin for the development of flavors (such as chocolate flavors) that contain cinnamates, and it is used for chocolate bars, ice cream, milk products, and syrups. In Denmark and Sweden, benzoin is popular as a flavoring for baked goods that contain vanilla or cassia, as it is used to fix these flavors and increase their spiciness. Other food uses include as a glazing agent, in syrups for turbidity, and as a chewing gum base (Japan) (Kashio and Johnson, 2001).

Benzoin has antiseptic, stimulant, expectorant, and diuretic properties medicinally. The national pharmacopoeias of Britain, China, France, Italy, Japan, Switzerland, Thailand, and the United States all contain specifications for benzoin. For lung problems, including coughs, laryngitis, bronchitis, and upper respiratory tract disorders, benzoin tincture is inhaled with steam. Several proprietary products also contain benzoin, such as lotions to prevent cold sores, a paint to treat warts (Compound Podophyllum Paint), and a mouthwash (Ondroly-A; in the Italian pharmacopoeia) for dental disorders, and an antibacterial powder for the skin (Purol; Indonesia) which uses Sumatra benzoin. Many over-the-counter herbal medicine preparations are becoming more common in Western society, including benzoin (Sumatra) for coughs and colds, and topical treatments for skin irritations, wounds, and ulcers. Benzoin is also becoming more prevalent in aromatherapy, being regarded as soothing and relaxing for muscles. Benzoin also has a long use in traditional Chinese medicine (listed in the Chinese pharmacopoeia), as it has been employed for restoring consciousness, increasing the blood flow, and as a pain medicament (Kashio and Johnson, 2001; Shin, 2003).

The largest volume of benzoin in the world is used for incense, and this is usually in the form of the Sumatra type. Benzoin is used in the religious worship of a number of major religions, including Muslim,

Hindu, Chinese Buddhist, and for mixtures used in the Catholic and Orthodox churches. Retail products, such as Ratus Dedes, a mixture of fragrant herbs and barks including benzoin in the form of a small golf ball, are sold in Indonesia for placing in open fires to exude fragrance, or for scenting young women's hair (Kashio and Johnson, 2001).

In India, benzoin is thought to be similar in quality to frankincense for burning in the temple in front of the deities Brahma, Vishnu, and Shiva. It also has a long medicinal use for respiratory support (especially for dry cough) and for skin conditions.

Known Chemical Constituents

The two types of benzoin have chemical differences that account for their organoleptic differences, and ultimately these differences also determine which applications the benzoin will be sold for on the market. Both are used for flavor and fragrance purposes, but the different grades are shipped to different areas of the market.

The resin is made up of mixtures of organic acids and esters, mostly two alcohols combined with cinnamic acid, and free cinnamonic and benzoic acids. Siam benzoin is characterized by benzoic acid and its esters (such as coniferyl benzoate, benzyl benzoate, and cinnamyl benzoate), whereas the Sumatra benzoin is characterized by cinnamic acid and its esters (such as coniferyl cinnamate and cinnamyl cinnamate). Vanillin is present in both types of benzoin and gives it a characteristic vanilla fragrance (especially in the Siam type). In an analysis of two different benzoin gums, Siam and Sumatra, the major components of the volatile oil fraction were found to be benzyl benzoate (76 to 80 percent for both oils), benzoic acid (12 percent), methyl benzoate (1 percent), allyl benzoate (1 percent for Siam), styrene (2 percent), cinnamic acid (3 percent), and benzyl cinnamate (3 percent for Sumatra) (Quezada, 2003; Kashio and Johnson, 2001; Fernandez et al., 2003; Nitta et al., 1984).

CAMPHOR: COOL AND CAMPHOROUS

Scientific name: *Cinnamomum camphora.*
Common name: Camphor.
Plant family: Lauraceae.

Origin: China, Japan, Korea, Taiwan, and other adjacent parts of East Asia. It grows mostly in mesic forests and on well-drained stream banks. In Australia the camphor tree has become naturalized, as well as in areas of the United States, such as along the Gulf Coast and in California. In the areas where it has naturalized it is now considered a noxious weed, as it is starting to replace native plants with its spread.

See Photo G.12 in the color photo gallery.

Camphor is a pure white powder that is said to look like wet snow. Synthetic camphor is also very common on the market. In Nepal, a relative plant called *sinkauli dhup* is sometimes used as a substitute for camphor.

Description of Plant

The camphor tree is a dense shiny-leaved tree that grows 50 to 150 feet tall and its branches can spread to twice that width. The foliage starts out a burgundy color and then turns to dark green. Each of the leaves have yellow veins. Inconspicuous flowers are produced in spring, followed by large crops of pea-sized berries that turn black with maturity. The tree is easily identified when crushing a leaf produces the distinctive camphor odor.

Historical and Current Usage

The camphor tree is considered a sacred tree. It is associated with the god Shiva, and its aroma is thought to be both pleasing and intoxicating. Camphor is mostly known in the Western world for its use in chest rub formulas for children who have colds and coughs, but it has a much deeper history of use as medicine, incense, and aroma. Although most people are familiar with its use in rub formulas, camphor can also be burned as an incense for treating colds.

Camphor's fragrance is strong and penetrating, and it has a pungent and bitter flavor. Camphor feels cool on the skin (similar to menthol), but it also produces a numbing effect, as well as irritating qualities. Camphor is used medicinally for treating many kinds of ailments, including parasitic infections and toothaches. Its uses that have been backed by science include as an antiseptic and as treatment for diarrhea, inflammation, itching, and nervous conditions.

In Nepal the camphor tree is used in various ways. The camphor itself is distilled from the flowers. An incense can also be obtained from the heartwood of the roots, and is considered to be very valuable. Camphor is regarded to be useful for purification, and able to purify the entire body. In this way, it is also used on the funeral pyres during cremations at Pashupatinath, VaranasiVarnasi, and in Southern India (Muller-Ebeling et al., 2000).

When someone is sick in Nepal and no healer, lama, or shaman is available, then a piece of camphor wood may be burned and prayed over, as it is said to be beneficial for the sick person. The shamans of Nepal also use camphor as a traveling herb, and invoke *kapur* in their mantras which is supposed to help them fly better (Muller-Ebeling et al., 2000).

Known Chemical Constituents

Camphor is a white crystalline solid ketone, with a characteristic odor and pungent taste and the chemical makeup of $C_{10}H_{16}O$. Since the natural camphor ("Japan camphor") is insufficient to meet the various market needs of camphor, it is widely synthesized from alpha-pinene obtained from turpentine. The natural form of camphor is produced by steam distillation of the wood of the camphor tree. About five different chemotypes of camphor trees exist with differing amounts of camphor, linalool, 1,8-cineole, nerolidol, and borneol. Certain chemotypes are favored for camphor extraction over others.

CEDAR: HELPING YOU TO FIND YOUR VISION

Scientific names: *Cedrus atlantic; Cedrus deodora; Calocedrus decurrens; Cedrus libani; Juniperus virginiana; Thuja occidentalis*

Common names: Atlantic cedar (North Africa); Himalayan cedar (Himalayas, India); Incense cedar;Cedar of Lebanon (Asia Minor); Red cedar; White Cedar

Plant family: Various; Pinaceae (Cedrus), Cupressaceae (*Calocedrus* and *Juniperus*)

Origin: Different kinds of cedars are found throughout the world, and a few species are indigenous to the United States. Sometimes Juniper species are referred to as cedar and used in a similar manner (red cedar).

See Photo G.13 in the color photo gallery.

Description of Plant

The typical cedar appearance is of a more or less conical evergreen with the characteristic bent branches (at the branch tips), giving the tree a graceful appearance. The raw product consists of the dried leaves (usually stripped from the evergreen, bladelike branches) or the wood.

Historical and Current Usage

"Cedar" used for incense use can be from one of several species of cedar trees or other evergreen species, such as Juniper and Calocedrus, depending on the location. Typically the local cedar tree species is the type that is used; however, differences exist in the aroma of the various species. For example, Native Americans use "cedar" frequently, and "flat cedar" or "incense cedar" *(Calocedrus decurrens)* may be used in the western United States for ceremony, while "Navaho Cedar" *(Juniperus* sp.) may be used in the southwest, depending on local availability and custom.

Cedar is one of the most important sacred herbs used by the Lakota and other Native Americans for ceremony. The importance and reason for its use by the Native Americans has been echoed by several unrelated cultures throughout the world. Cedar is for the aid of visions and for helping the body and mind in times of great spiritual anxiety and stress. Furthermore, it is used by the Native Americans for discovering one's "purpose" in life, and how to find one's path in life to walk in beauty and help people and the earth along the way.

According to Chief Phil Crazybull, a medicine man and chief of the Lakota, cedar is used not only in ceremony but also in homes, because it helps to create good dreams and visions during sleep. He explains,

> The spirits of the energy of cedar come from our ancestral way because Turtle Island (the Earth) was born with cedar on it, and because of this it is one of the oldest medicines that we have, and so it is one of the most simplest and the most powerful because it is so old.

In addition to the use of cedarwood for incense, cedarwood is well known for its aromatic and insect-repelling properties. For this reason, pet bedding is lined with cedar shavings, and cedar blocks are sometimes inserted into clothes drawers to keep out moths. Native Americans use a box made of cedarwood in which to keep sacred feathers, which are also used to fan incense smoke.

In the ancient world of Mesopotamia, according to Susanne Fischer-Rizzi (1996), the cedar of Lebanon was revered for use in ritual cleansing, and its form signified qualities that were sought after in those times: strength, dignity, power, and vitality. Cedar is used in many cultures for its ability to help us reflect and meditate for the right answer to difficult problems, for aid in clearing our breathing, and to help us to create vivid and prophetic dreams (Fischer-Rizzi, 1996).

In the Himalayas, the cedar forests are said to be among the most beautiful and majestic forests of the world. The Himalayan cedar *(Cedrus deodora)* appears itself as a strong-looking tree, with fringes of delicacy, as the tips of the branches and the top of the tree flop over at the top. Its gray-green appearance seems to add wisdom and timelessness to the tree, and its cones are like wood-crafted roses. The Himalayas themselves are a powerful mountain range, considered by the local inhabitants to be the "seat of the gods." They contain the powerful contrast of high, rugged mountaintops that are bare and rocky, topped only by the most resilient of plant species, such as mugwort and juniper, and the southern deep valleys that are home to monsoon-drenched forests with ferns and tall scarlet rhododendron. The scent and power of the Himalayan incense plants often bring clarity and an expansiveness derived from their place of origin (Fischer-Rizzi, 1996).

In ancient Egypt the burning of twigs and fine shavings of cedarwood was common practice. Cedar oil was also used in embalming practices, and often cedar branches and wood would be included in the burial of kings (Fischer-Rizzi, 1996).

Known Chemical Constituents

Cedar leaf oil, also called Thuja oil, is obtained by the steam distillation of the fresh leaves of the cedar, most commonly *Thuja occidentalis*. Branches and leaves contain about 0.3 to 1.0 percent oil. Major components are d-a-pinene, d-a-thujone, 1-fechone, 1-borneal, and acetic-, formic- and isovaleric-acids.

Cedarwood oil is a mixture of volatile sesquiterpenes from the heartwood of *Cedrus,* as well as other plants commonly used to extract "cedarwood oil," such as *Juniperus* and *Cupressus* species. In fact, the *Juniperus* and *Cupressus* species are used more commonly for the production of cedarwood oil because they have the highest yield. However, cedar species are still used for the production of cedarwood oil, such as *Cedrus atlantica* and *C. deodara.* Typical sesquiterpene content of cedarwood oil includes alpha- and beta-cedrene, thujopsene, cuparene, cedrol, and widdrol (Langenheim, 2004; Fischer-Rizzi, 1996).

COPAL: LATIN AMERICAN FOOD OF THE GODS

Scientific names: *Guibourtia demeusei; Agathis dammara* or *A. alba; Canarium Bengalese; Vateria indica; Hymenaea verrucosa; Agathis australis; Hymenaea verrucosa.*

Common names: *Congo copal;* Manila copal;East Indian copal; Indian copal; Zanzibar copal (eastern Africa); Kauri copal(New Zealand); Madagascar copal (Rai, 1981; Case et al., 2003).

Plant Family: Mostly Burseraceae.

Origin: *Protium copal* is a subcanopy tree that grows in a range of environments, from primary forests to deciduous secondary forests from Mexico, Guatemala, and Belize. The word *copal* was borrowed by the Maya from the Aztecs word *copalli.* Not to be confused with *Copaifera* (Copaiba balsam), which is from western Africa.

See Photos G.14 and G.15 in the color photo gallery.

The common name *copal* has produced much confusion, as several tree species are thought to produce a type of "copal." The discussion here will focus on *Protium copal,* but *Bursera* species are also considered a primary source of copal from Mesoamerica. Another genus that is a source of popular copal is *Hymenaea,* of which two very similar species exist, one in South America, and the other in Africa. Although the various copal types are derived from different species, they are also distinguished by harvesting technique.

The three main appearances of copal resin on the American market are black *(copal negro),* golden *(copal oro),* and white *(copal blanco).*

These copals can come from various tree species, and it usually depends on the region of sale. A "frankincense of the gods" mixture exists in which all three types are mixed together. Although the three types of copal can usually be distinguished by color, chemical analytical techniques can be used to tell them apart. In recent analyses, calcium carbonate was found as an included ingredient as a possible whitener (Fischer-Rizzi, 1996; Case et al., 2003; Edwards and Moens, 2003).

Description of Plant

The *Protium copal* tree is a small subcanopy tree, with smooth, tan-brown bark. The trunk is generally thin (about ten centimeters), with long branches that produce a thin, leggy crown. The tree produces inconspicuous flowers and larger attractive fruits that have been found on the tree at all times during the year.

Historical and Current Usage

Copal has an ancient history of use in Latin and South America, especially in the Maya, Inca, and Aztec territories in Mexico and Peru. In these cultures, incense use was integral to the medicine system, as well as for divine worship and for magical ceremonies. Fragrant plants, which were plentiful in the jungle, were particularly thought to possess a great amount of power and were not only able to heal, but also to cleanse the body of its spiritual impurities. Copal to these cultures was among the most important of the incense-burning substances.

According to the holy book of the Maya, the earth god took copal from the tree of life and gifted it to the Mayan culture. Incense use in general has and continues to be important in the Mayan culture, as censers have been found that date back to 600 BC. The use of copal by the Maya has two main aspects. First, the incense is seen to be essential in maintaining relationships with and promoting the action of some deities and ancestors. Second, the incense smoke is thought to kick off a transformative process that was held by the Maya's religious and cosmological belief. The Maya also see the incense as a "food of the gods," as both maize and copal are connected with this ritual understanding. Copal, in ancient times as well as today, has been found shaped in the form of maize and tortillas, and as small disks called pesos that look similar to coins. The "pesos" have been offered as a sort of sacrificial money to the gods in return for a prayer being answered, such as a good hunt. The Inca considered copal to be special for the god of the sun, and in this god's reverence it was burned four times a day (Langenheim, 2004; Fischer-Rizzi, 1996).

The South and Central American copal is either yellow/white, transparent, or black, and each has a different aroma. The transparent variety is lighter, fruitier, and a little lemony, and is used in spiritual, cleansing, and cognitive work. The black copal, sometimes referred to as night copal, is generally thought to be more powerful and mystical, possessing a heavy balsamic aroma, and is thought to be good for grounding and aiding the soul in healing in its darkest areas. Although originally from the Americas, "copal" resins can be found on the market from scattered areas of the world, including Africa, India, Madagascar, and the Philippines, Indian copal is derived from the tree *Vateria indica* (Rai, 1981). Congo copal is mostly used in varnish and paint manufacturing. Manila copal is known to be an important source of cash income for indigenous collectors in Southeast Asia (Fischer-Rizzi, 1996; Quezada, 2003; Conelly, 1985).

Copal has been important in traditional medicine for treating respiratory and dental problems, and for its vermifuge and antiparasitic properties. Today copal is best known for its use as an incense in Mayan and Catholic ceremonies, especially where copal naturally occurs. In addition, copal has found its way into the widespread practice of the sweat lodge ceremony, which plays an important part in reviving Native American traditions, as well as in traditional forms of dancing at powwows, such as the Aztec dances.

Before the Aztec dances begin, a vessel with smoldering copal will be offered to each of the four directions. With special respect and reverence given to the four directions and the four elements, the Aztec dancers give a soulful performance decorated with showy feathers. Some dancers may wear headdresses with feathers that are five feet tall. This occurs while the sweet smell of copal and the beats of drums waft through the air.

Mexican copal has been reported to be used as a vaginal contraceptive (water extract of stems and leaves), and has been verified in experimental investigations to have sperm aggregatory activity. In this case it was found that the proteins present in the extract cause aggregation of sperm heads (Serrano and Garcia-Suarez, 2001).

Bursera species are also considered a main source of copal in Mesoamerica, and the genus *Bursera* is considered the New World relative of frankincense and myrrh (*Boswellia* and *Commiphora*). *B. pinnata* may be a prevalent source of copal because it is commonly found growing as a fencerow tree and therefore it is abundant (Langenheim, 2004).

According to Rufino Paxi, a shaman of the Ayamara of the Andean high plains in Bolivia, incense is used as an offering to the spirits both in the house and outdoors. He says copal is among the safest of the incenses and can be easily used indoors and even imbibed. When a person is sick from altitude in Bolivia, copal may be mashed with wine to help the person get better. He says that copal can be used to cense money for bringing good fortune, and for the clothes to bring the spirit of money. Rufino says (Paxi, Personal Communication, May 22, 2004),

> Copal is bought by the pounds and kilos and we pulverize it in the house. Once pulverized you can use it any time you need—either in the night or the day—it doesn't matter. Copal is used to relate and to be able to communicate with nature and the universe. Copal is like a food for the [spirit of the] animals and all the materials we want and the plants as well. [Also it is good] for clothing and money. [Copal is good] for the house that is like a mother as well. It is the smoke that gives us good vibes. For the houses, the houses are like mothers and should always be given copal. Also agricultural products are given copal. [Copal is] good and beneficial for humanity.

Known Chemical Constituents

Bursera species are characterized by a dominance of mono- and sesquiterpenes. However, many of the species contain mixtures of as much as twenty-five compounds, including the terpenes. One predominant compound is found in some species, such as ß-phellandrene or ß-myrcene. The essential oil from *copal blanco* (probably from *Bursera pinnata*) is mainly alpha-copaene (approximately 15 percent) and germacrene (14 percent); *copal oro* (probably from *Hymenaea courbaril*) is dominated by alpha-pinene (21 percent) and limonene (26 percent); and *copal negro* (probably from

Protium copal) is alpha-pinene (18 percent), sabinene (13 percent), and limonene (17 percent) (Case et al., 2003).

DRAGON'S BLOOD: SMOKE FROM THE DRAGON

Scientific names: *Daemenorops draco* B.L. and about nine other *Daemenorops* spp.; *Dracaena draco* L. (Warning: several red-sapped plant products have the common name of dragon's blood, including *Croton lechlerii.*); *Dracaena cochinchinensis; Dracaena cinnabari.*

Common names: Dragon's blood; Chinese dragon's blood.

Plant family: Palmae *(Daemonorops)* and Dracaenaceae *(Dracaena)*.

Origin: Dragon's blood is the common name for the resin from several different plant species, and not all have similar uses (Pearson et al., 2001). Dragon's blood comes from the marsh regions of Southeast Asia, Java, Borneo, Sumatra, and the Moluccan islands (Fischer-Rizzi, 1996). *Dracaena draco* is indigenous to the Canary Islands. *Dracaena draco* is originally from the Canary Islands, and during the fifteenth century it was a very valuable product of the early explorers (Langenheim, 2004).

See Photo G.16 in the color photo gallery.

Dragon's blood incense resin is a red resin that is collected, cleansed, and dried from the fruit of the dragon's blood liana (*Daemonorops* spp.). It is sold on the market either as pellets or on sticks.

Dragon's blood (from *Daemonorops draco*) has been found sold with other drugs of abuse, but its abuse potential alone has been found to be minimal, as it had no observable abuse-related effects in mice (Ford et al., 2001).

Description of Plant

Daemonorops is a genus of lianas that produces about nine species from the Indomalesianrain forest that are used as the source of the main dragon's blood in commerce. These lianas produce little scaly fruits that seep a red resin between the scales, which is used as incense. The *Dracena draco* palm is a stout and prehistoric-looking tree with thick branches and short palm leaves. It is extremely slow growing, taking ten to fifteen years to grow two to three feet. The crown is divided by several branches, and is referred to as a "multi-headed dragon."

Historical and Current Usage

Dragon's blood incense is believed to be cleansing, and can be used for clearing negative energies and for protection. It may be used in sacrifices in rituals in India, or may be used with a frankincense mixture in churches, as it has many of the same spiritual and cleansing properties (Fischer-Rizzi, 1996).

Dragon's blood from *Dracaena cinnabari* is the basis for several myths, such as that by Pliny, which attribute the resin's creation to a battle between a dragonlike creature and an elephant. The mixing of the blood of the two animals was said to produce the resin. Another Greek myth, The eleventh labor of Hercules: The apples of the Hespérides, referred to a hundred-headed dragon that was the guardian of the nymph daughters *(Hesperides)* of Atlas, the titan who holds up heaven and earth. The dragon is killed by either Hercules or Atlas (depending on the version), and the dragon's blood flowed through the land, giving rise to dragon's blood trees. This form of dragon's blood was treasured by the Greeks, Romans, and Arabs for its magical and medicinal properties.

Many traditional uses exist for *Daemonorops* resin. With its astringent qualities it is used as an eyewash, for dental health and washes, and for diarrhea and dysentery. It also has proven antimicrobial activity, and is used as a pigment for tinting toothpastes, imitation tortoise-shell, marble, and varnishes. It was also used to tint violins in the eighth century (Langenheim, 2004).

Aromatic compounds from dragon's blood resin are known to exhibit antifungal activity (Wang et al., 1995). Studies on the carcinogenicity of various isoflavonoids and flavonoids from dragon's blood resin found that the majority of these compounds poses none or very little potential carcinogenic activity (Vachalkova et al., 1995).

Dragon's blood (from *Dracaena*) is used as a varnish and for photo engraving. It was highly valued in trade in the fifteenth century. The early inhabitants of the Canary Islands also used dragon's blood resin, as was evidenced by cave drawings there. (Langenheim, 2004; Quezada, 2003).

Known Chemical Constituents

Daemonorops dragon's blood (the main kind in commerce) consists of the well-known red pigments, dracorhodin and dracorubin, and more than 50 percent of the resin alcohol, as dracoresinotannol, which is related to benzoic and benzoyl acetic acids. The resin is made up mostly of phenolic compounds, although diterpene resin acids have also been described. Other compounds present include benzoyl acetic ester, dracoresene, dracoalban, and cinnamic acids. In addition, six A-types of flavonoid deoxyproanthocyanidins have also been found in *Daemonorops* resin (Langenheim, 2004).

Dragon's blood resin is known to contain various isoflavonoids and flavonoids. *Dracena draco* was analyzed and found to contain twenty-one different phenolic compounds in its resin. *Dracena draco* subsp. *draco* and subsp. *ajgal* and *D. tamaranae* all contain the major flavonoid constituent of (2S)-4,7'-dihyroxy-8-methylflavan (Vachalkova et al., 1995; Gonzalez et al., 2004).

Dracaena cochinchinensis from the Yunnan province of China was found to contain the aromatic compounds ethyl-p-hydroxy benzoate, 7,4'-dihydroxyflavan, 7-hydroxy-4'-methoxyflavan, 7,4'-dihydroxyflavone, and lourerin as well as a known steroid saponin (Wang et al., 1995). *Dracaena cinnabari* was found to contain numerous flavonoids, the biflavonoids 2'-methoxysocotrin-5'-ol, socotrin-4'-ol, homoisosocotrin-4'-ol, a new biflavonoid called cinnabarone, a new triflavonoid called damalachawin, various triterpenoids, and sterols (Masaoud, Himmelreich, et al., 1995; Himmelreich et al., 1995; Masaoud, Ripperger, Himmelreich, et al., 1995; Masaoud, Ripperger, Porzel, et al., 1995; Masaoud, Schmidt, et al., 1995). In the Chinese dragon's blood, nine chalcones were isolated and elucidated, including a new one called cochinchinenin (Zhou et al., 2001). When several types of Chinese dragon's blood resin were examined, they were all found to have similar chemical constituents, whereas the imported resin was found to be different (Wang et al., 1995).

It has been shown that fungal associations or attack on *Dracaena chochinchinensis* are able to increase the production and yield of dragon's blood resin (by about 66 to 120 percent), but the exact role these fungi play in production of resin and resin quality is still unknown (Jiang et al., 1995).

EUCALYPTUS: BEATS THE TOXINS OUT OF YOU

Scientific names: *Eucalyptus* spp. several species are used for the essential oil and incense, especially *E. citriodora* (lemon-scented gum) and *E. globulus* (blue gum).

Common names: *Eucalyptus* species are usually referred to as eucalyptus or sometimes various types of "gums."

Plant family: Myrtaceae.

Origin: Originally from Australia, and now cultivated all over the world.

See Photo G.17 in the color photo gallery.

Most *Eucalyptus* species are tall trees, and are among the tallest in the world. Characteristic of the eucalyptus is the scent, which many people know due to the widespread cultivation of the tree. The trees are native to Australia and have been used for a long time by the aboriginal people. Characteristic features of eucalyptus are that they are fast growing trees with bark that peels from the trunk and falls to the ground. The leaves may be shaped in various ways, but are often long lanceolate leaves or oval.

Historical and Current Usage

Eucalyptus leaves may be burned as a fumigant and as incense. They may be used fresh or dry, and the essential oil is also used for making incense sticks and cones. The aboriginal people of Australia are known to use eucalyptus in many ways, including as food, medicines, as timber for general construction, poles, tools, canoes, and bowls. As eucalyptus has spread around the world, many other traditional cultures have adapted to using it for various medicinal applications. Medicinal applications include as an antiseptic, for colds and lung problems, and topically for ulcers, wounds, and other skin problems. Eucalyptus is also used as a fumigant or incense, and the leaves are also sometimes heated so that their steam can be inhaled as an antiseptic and to treat lung problems and colds (Morton, 1981).

Eucalyptus oils and the branches are also used often in steam and dry air saunas. The eucalyptus oils are either placed over the rocks, or may be used in a tapotement treatment in which eucalyptus branches are tapped (or beaten) over the body. In Russia, it is quite common to find in the bathhouses a ritual in which people take turns beating each other with eucalyptus branches. On occasion, eucalyptus leaves are also used in sweat lodges by Native Americans for treating a fever (Okugawa et al., 1996).

Eucalyptus is also favored in perfumery, and the lemon gum produces a lemon-scented oil that is rich in citronellal. Kenyans also favor a honey that is produced from this species (Watt and Breyer-Brandwijk, 1962).

Most people in the Western world are familiar with eucalyptus, since it has been naturalized to so many places around the world, and because of its distinctive scent. Eucalyptus essential oil has been proven to have antibacterial activity (Dodia, 2004; Bartynska and Budzikur-Ramza, 2001; Pattnaik et al., 1996; Scala et al., 2001). However, large doses of the oil can be toxic, and the citronellal that is in eucalyptus has been found to be mutagenic.

Known Chemical Constituents

The bark of eucalyptus may contain up to 12 percent tannin. The major component of eucalyptus oil is 1,8-cineole. Myrtillin is present in the leaf and its extract, which possesses hyperglycemic activity. In the leaves of *E. citradora,* betulinic and ursolic acids, eucalyptin, and ß-sitosterol are present. The oil in the glabrous leaves has been reported to be 65.5 percent citronellal, 12.2 percent citronellol, and 3.5 percentisopulegol. Leaves that are hairy have been reported to hold a higher content of oil (Atal and Kapur, 1982).

FRANKINCENSE: THE CHOICE INCENSE

Scientific names: *Boswellia serrata* (and other *Boswellia* spp.).
Common names: Olibanum, boswellia.
Plant family: Burseraceae.
Origin: Several species of Boswellia provide the incense product called frankincense. The botanical knowledge of the species of *Boswellia* providing frankincense is still inadequate, and several of the species are thought to have gone extinct or nearly extinct. In ancient times, *B. papyrifera* was thought to be mainly used for deriving frankincense, and in classical times it was thought to be *B. sacra,* but today frankincense is derived mostly from *B. carteri, B. frereana,* and

B. serrata (Tucker, 1986). Frankincense species are cultivated in India and Africa, especially Somalia and Ethiopia.

See Photo G.18 in the color photo gallery.

Description of Plant

Frankincense trees reach only about twenty feet in height, have a distinct gnarly and rough appearance, and grow in rocky, dry soil. The "frankincense belt" is a narrow (about nine miles) strip of land that has a specific soil type that the trees like to grow in, and the main frankincense tree that comes from this area is *B. carteri*. Of the twenty-five types of frankincense that used to be available, only about three are now known and available on the market.

Historical and Current Usage

Frankincense is an archaic term for "choice incense." Frankincense is a dried resin that is gold in color. Sometimes when frankincense is used in mixtures it is coated with a bronze color for its visual effect. Frankincense and myrrh are two classical incenses that are among the most used and included in several spirituals traditions. Frankincense and myrrh are also thought of as companions, and are often burned together. Along with this symbolism, frankincense is thought of as providing male energy, and myrrh the female. In classical times, frankincense resin was as valuable as gold.

Frankincense is often thought of in terms of Christian spirituality since it was brought as a gift to baby Jesus by the Magi, was one of the eight pleasing fragrances of Moses, and is mentioned in the Bible many times. Still today it is used in Roman Catholic worship, as well as in other denominations throughout the world.

Frankincense and other incense resins were traded from the southern coast of Arabian Peninsula for more than a millennium. At this time, Arabia was known as happy Arabia, because great wealth was gained due to this trade. Many believe that it is the Egyptians who first began the trade in incenses. The Babylonians, Sumerians, and Assyrians also were known to love incense, but it is not known whether they were using frankincense and myrrh or local plants and resins. The Egyptians offered incense to the gods as a sacrifice—a "food of the gods," since the gods were thought to starve without it. Incense was also used in sacrifices, to drive away evil spirits, to honor a person, and during important festivities and celebrations. The Egyptians and Persians considered the right to offer incense something that belonged only to the priesthood (including kings); however, the Greeks and Romans considered incense offering not only a right but also a duty by everyone. The harvesting of frankincense was also something that was to be done only by certain appointed families, and because it was regarded as divine no impure acts were allowed by the harvesters (Langenheim, 2004).

Even though many other fragrances became known to the Greeks, as in Egypt frankincense and myrrh remained the most highly regarded incenses, and were commonly burned to worship the gods. In fact, almost all of the plants from Arabia used for incense burning became well known in Greece, Egypt, Crete, and Mesopotamia. It was thought that the two together, myrrh and frankincense, were perfect for reaching the heavens (Fischer-Rizzi, 1996).

In the classical times of the Greeks and Romans, frankincense was believed to have originated in a story of love, as was myrrh. In this story, the Sun seduces a king's daughter, and upon discovering this the king kills and buries his daughter. The Sun sought the dead girl and tried to revive her unsuccessfully with his warm rays. However, the Sun promises the dead girl that she can still come up to him in the sky, so he covers her body with a fragrant nectar that then melts away up into the sky and fills the earth with its fragrance. It is said that the spot where her body laid is where the first shrub of frankincense rose slowly from the earth (Classen et al., 1994).

Frankincense is considered to have the powerful ability to not only cleanse the air of unpleasant smell, but also of negative energies. In this sense it may be burned in areas where the air seems thick and stuffy, or where people have argued, or a bad situation has occurred. For millennia it has been regarded as a way for aiding the human spirit that wants to remain open to the divine, and in communicating with heavenly or spiritual energies (Fischer-Rizzi, 1996).

Frankincense resin has been used not only for spiritual purposes, but also for medicinal reasons, as even today it is known as a popular and clinically validated treatment for rheumatism and osteoarthritis (Kimmatkar et al., 2003). It is also known to reduce stress and muscle tension (Fischer-Rizzi, 1996). Frankincense is used internally to treat inflammatory conditions, especially for joint pain and sports recovery. Frankincense is also known to be wound healing, and a disinfectant, and when it is burned indoors in areas such as churches it is believed to protect against infectious diseases and negative influences. This was especially important when pilgrims slept in churches and the "gifts" received were perishable goods, and when pestilence was a more frequently encountered problem. In addition, as far back as Egyptian times farmers have been known to fumigate wheat with frankincense in order to keep moths away (Fischer-Rizzi, 1996; Reichling et al., 2004).

One interesting effect that frankincense has is on the human voice. Recently researchers found that the voice carried better after the air had been exposed to frankincense. This may have been another reason why frankincense was used in churches during a sermon (Fischer-Rizzi, 1996).

In Islam, among the teachings of the Prophet, frankincense is

> warming in the second degree, desiccative in the first, and contains slight costiveness. It is very beneficial, and has little harm. Among its benefits is that it is useful for hemorrhages, for stomach winds, and clears ulcers of the eye, causes flesh to grow on most ulcers, strengthens and warms the weak stomach, dries up phlegm, dries moistures of the chest, clears darkness of the sight and prevents foul ulcers from spreading. Used as a fumigant (incense), it is beneficial for pestilence and sweetens the smell of the air. (Johnson, 1998, pp. 271-272)

When referring to the sweetness of the air, this is an important quality that goes beyond just aroma for the sake of pleasure—it implies that sweetness drives away evil and attracts angels. It is also thought to be good for forgetfulness (Johnson, 1998).

In Egypt, frankincense was a favorite among the Egyptians' highly developed art of incense use. According to legend, the bird Phoenix brought frankincense to the Egyptians, and it was thought to be a gift directly from the gods. Frankincense was also an important ingredient in *kyphi,* the most favored of the Egyptian incense mixtures that was not only used throughout Egypt but was also exported (Fischer-Rizzi, 1996).

In Mesopotamia, the word for frankincense was identical to that for Lebanon cedar, and it was this substance that was used as frankincense to be burned on the altars of Baal-Marduk, and it was one of the most favored of all the incenses (Fischer-Rizzi, 1996).

Research has found that the sesquiterpenes present in frankincense may increase the oxygen levels in the brain by 28 percent, which undoubtedly may produce other benefits in the body, such as an increase in the activity of the hypothalamus—and its subsequent effect on emotions, learning, and attitude—and improving immune function, hormone balance, and energy levels (Williams, 2004).

Pure frankincense is available in different qualities, including frankincense Eritrea, pellets temperament, light powder, and first choice. Aden frankincense, Somalia first quality (or Mushaad), and Oman first quality are highly recommended. Many mixtures of frankincense are sold with various names, including the Three-King Mixture, Spice Mixture, Precious Mixture, Colorful Mixture, Light Arabian Pontificate, Palestine King, Black Lourdes, Gloria, and Angelus (Fischer-Rizzi, 1996).

The frankincense that is used today in Catholic churches has been reported to be often a mixture of balsams: 66 percent frankincense, 27 percent benzoin, and 7 percent storax (Langenheim, 2004). Sophisticated chemical analyses have been developed, such as high performance liquid chromatography (HPLC), in order to distinguish between frankincense of different origins and species (Buechele et al., 2003).

Known Chemical Constituents

Alpha-pinene is thought to be one of the main compounds contributing to frankincense's characteristic fresh and balsamic odor, with gamma-butyrolactones lending strong coumarinic odors. The volatile components of *Boswellia serrata* essential oil have been found to be about thirty-five different chemical constituents of which alpha-pinene (73 percent) was the predominant constituent. Other monoterpenoids include beta-pinene (2.05 percent), cis-verbenol (1.97 percent), trans-pinocarveol (1.80 percent), borneol (1.78 percent), myrcene (1.71 percent), verbenone (1.71 percent), limonene (1.42 percent), thuja-2,4(10)-diene (1.18 percent) and p-cymene (1.0 percent). One sesquiterpene, alpha-copaene (0.13 percent), has been identified in the essential oil (Kasali et al., 2002).

Boswellia serrata has been found to have anti-inflammatory, antiallergic, and immunomodulating activity due to its content of boswellic acids (pentacyclic triterpenes). Boswellic acids act as specific, noncompetitive, nonredox inhibitors of a key enzyme (5-lipoxy-genase) for biosynthesizing leukotrienes (Pungle et al., 2003).

MUGWORT AND MOXA: PROTECTION AND MEDICINE WORLDWIDE

Scientific names: *Artemisia vulgaris,* including other *Artemisia* species, possibly *A.chinense* (syn. *C. artemisiodes* and *C. chinense*). Some confusion exists on the market regarding which species are used as mugwort and which are used for moxa. Artemisia is also sold sometimes erroneously as "sage" for incense use, although a California native *Artemisia* is commonly called California sagebrush.

Common names: moxa, wormwood, sage.

Plant family: Asteraceae.

Origin: Mugwort is an introduced plant to many areas of the world, including the United States, Europe, and China, because it adapts and naturalizes quickly.

See Photo 1.4 in Chapter 1 and Photo G.19 in the color photo gallery.

Mugwort may be prepared several different ways. Most commonly just the leaves or the leaves and the stems are harvested, dried, and then prepared into loose dry leaves, a smudge stick, or moxa cones or sticks.

Description of Plant

Many species of *Artemisia* exist. This discussion will focus on *A. vulgaris. Artemisia* species tend to be highly aromatic and have characteristic grayish-green or silvery leaves. Mugwort is a grayish-green, shrubby or herbaceous plant that has long stems with oval-shaped or often forked (in three lobes) leaves.

Historical and Current Usage

Mugwort has been used by many cultures throughout the world as an incense, for medicine, and for superstitious and magical purposes. Almost everywhere it is found it is known for its use in healing, divination, and for aiding in dreams and visions. Many people who live in the United States and are used to hiking in places with poison oak are sure to have heard the folkloric use of mugwort, which often grows among the poison oak. It is the case of an antidote living among the poison that is so often found in the botanical world. When exposed to poison oak, the rubbing of mugwort leaves on the affected areas is said to prevent the rash caused by the poison oak. It is also a common folkloric antidote to snakebite in many cultures (Garg, 2000-2001), and rubbing it on the skin is supposed to also prevent leeches from attaching (Muller-Ebeling et al., 2000). Mugwort as an herb, however, has many other traditional medicinal uses, such as for bringing on menstruation, and topically for pruritis skin lesions (Tezuka et al., 1993). Mugwort is combusted for various healing and magic uses, as well as more mundane purposes, such as for its insect-repelling capability (Hwang et al., 1985).

In European herb lore, mugwort is also known as cronewort, as it is said to grow at the front doors of healers, and to be a favorite among them. Among the Native American community, it is used sometimes with the sweat lodge ceremony, bundled as a smudge stick or used as loose leaves, and burned before and during the sweat or in the water that is prepared for pouring on the stones (McCampbell, 2002).

Mugwort is considered by many as the most ancient incense of humankind. In Nepal, it is the most important of the herbaceous or leafy incense plants. It is used in various ways, and may be burned over heated limestone, placed on altars, hung in the house, or even rubbed on a shaman's drum for protection. In this part of the world mugwort is considered a traveling herb, as its seeds are used to put shamans in trances, and also to bring them back. A preblended incense made primarily of mugwort is available in the incense market, and used by the lamas of Nepal (Muller-Ebeling et al., 2000).

Mugwort is also known as "moxa" for the act of moxibustion in traditional Chinese medicine (TCM), and is often used by acupuncturists. Moxa has been used in TCM for more than 5,000 years, not only for the treatment of medical conditions, but also for their prevention. Originally, TCM was used only for the emperors of China and their court, but eventually the Chinese public demanded that these secrets of health and longevity be made available to the public. Although many herbs are used, and several are even combusted or heated in the practice of TCM, no other herb performs a similar function to moxa. It has the qualities of being able to clear obstructed energy in the energy channels of the body, and it has a calming effect that is sometimes used to enhance meditation. In addition, moxa is sometimes prepared as a liquid extract and used internally. Moxa has even been proven in double-blind, placebo-controlled studies for correcting certain health conditions, such as correcting the breech presentation of a fetus before birth (by stimulating acupoint BL 67 with moxa) (Cardini and Weixin, 1998).

Moxa is used in three basic ways. One preparation of moxa uses the "wool" from the hairy stems and leaves, which is shaped into a cone (available in different sizes). These cones are then used with either direct or indirect contact with the skin. According to Dr. Ira Golchehreh, a licensed acupuncturist and practitioner of TCM in San Rafael, California, an example of when moxa might be used directly on the skin would be for certain lung conditions, such as asthma. The moxa cone would be burned directly on the skin over the corresponding meridian to the lungs. However, Dr. Ira says this is very rarely done in the United States because few Americans would tolerate the procedure. He explains that in the TCM that is practiced in America, other, more appropriate, techniques are used. For indirect use with the skin, these cones are burned atop of what is called an "insulation," which is either a slice of garlic or ginger, or salt overtop of a particular meridian. The moxa on top of ginger is used in certain spleen or stomach conditions, and for joint pain. The moxa on top of garlic may be used for snakebites or certain skin infections, and an example of the moxa on top of salt is for stopping diarrhea (Dr. Ira Golcehreh, personal communication, March 2004).

Another main preparation of moxa is in the form of sticks, in which the dried leaves are rolled into a cigarlike stick. Dr. Ira says that these are never used with people with asthma or bronchial conditions so that the smoke does not aggravate their condition. They are used for diseases that are characterized in TCM as being "cold diseases," such as for viral infections. Dr. Ira says this is also the application that is most easily performed as self-care, if the person knows the nature of their illness and how to apply the moxa. For example, for runny noses, Dr. Ira says a person may light the end of the stick and blow it out, so that there is no flame, but there is a smoldering end. The smoldering end can be run about an inch or more from the skin along the areas of the face where the sinuses lie (the nose region and on top of the eyebrows). Dr. Ira noted that a person must take care not to drop ash on the skin, and he says that if this is done three times a day the sinuses will remain clear (Dr. Ira Golcehreh, personal communication, March 2004).

Another condition for which moxa may be used for self-care, according to Dr. Ira, is for cold sores around the mouth. First, ice should be run along the gums of the mouth and inside the inner part of the lips to cool them down. Then the lighted moxa stick may be slowly passed over the cold sore (without touching it) (Dr. Ira Golcehreh, personal communication, March 2004).

The third type of application for which moxa may be used is for the warming of the needles during acupuncture. Dr. Ira says that this is a technique that only a well-trained acupuncturist should use (not for self-care), and he added that many times in the United States this technique is not used because of the danger of ash dropping onto the skin. In his practice, he has replaced this technique with the use of modern moxa-containing lamps. As the patient undergoes acupuncture, he orients these specialized heat-producing lamps that are coated with moxa and other herbs near the areas of the skin that are being pierced, and allows the person to relax under the heat lamps for a while (Dr. Ira Golcehreh, personal communication, March 2004).

According to Myogen Steve Stucky, a Soto Zen priest of Rohnert Park, California, moxa is used for certain types of Buddhist ritual, such as during ordination in Chinese Buddhist sects:

> During these ordinations, three moxa cones are burned down to the skin on top of the monk's or nun's shaved head, overtop of the crown area. In these cases you can see that some Chinese Buddhist priests have these three scars on top of their head as a mark of taking their religious vows. The significance of the number three would be the vow to "take refuge in Buddha, Dharma, and Sangha," known as the Three Treasures of Buddhism. (Steve Stucky, personal communication, March 2004)

Known Chemical Constituents

The principal compounds in mugwort are total hydroxycinnamic acids (6 to 9 percent), chlorogenic acid (0.79 to 1.35 percent), 1,5-dicaffeoylquinic acid (0.51 to 1.25 percent), and 3,5-dicaffeoylquinic acid (2.2 to 2.6 percent) (Fraisse et al., 2003). Some of the flavonoids in mugwort are tricine, jaceosidine, eupafolin, chrysoeriol, diosmetin, homoeriodictyol, isorhamnetin, apigenin, eriodictyol, luteolin, luteolin 7-glucoside, kaempferol 3-glucoside, kaempferol 7-glucoside, kaempferol 3-rhamnoside, kaempferol 3-rutinoside, quercetin 3-glucoside, quercetin 3-galactoside, quercetin, rutin, and vitexin (Lee et al., 1998). Mono- and sesquiterpenes are the main compounds present in the essential oil of the blossom, with sabinene as the major chemical constituent in most cases, but in certain planting schemes this may be camphor (Bagchi et al., 2003; Michaelis et al., 1982). Essential oil from Croatia is known to be richer in hydrocarbons, and the plants to have a higher essential oil yield (0.09 to 0.61 percent) than French essential oil (0.04 to 0.15 percent) (Jerkovic et al., 2003).

MYRRH: THE FEMALE QUALITY OF INCENSE

Scientific names: Most commonly *Commiphora wightii* (Syn. *C. mukul*) and *C. myrrha* (Syn. *C. molmol*). Myrrh from the Bible is probably *C. erthraea, C. guidotii,* and/or *C. foliacea; C. abyssinica, C. schimperi, C. tenuis; C. madagascariensis; Myrrhis odorata; C. guidotii; C. guidotii; Cistus ladanifer.*

Common names: Myrrh; Abyssinian myrrh; Garden myrrh; Mecca myrrh; Scented myrrh; Myrrh of Genesis.

Plant family: Burseraceae.

Origin: *C. myrrha* is indigenous from northeast Africa to the Arabian world. *C. mukul* is indigenous to India. Although the predominately used myrrh today is *C. myrrha, C. erthraea* was thought to be the principal source of myrrh in ancient and classical times (Tucker, 1986).

See Photos G.20 and G.21 in the color photo gallery.

Description of Plant

Although the myrrh genus is diverse, the common myrrh tree grows in similar conditions and has a similar stunted, gnarly appearance as frankincense. Myrrh is a shrub or tree that grows to approximately thirty-three feet with a twelve-inch circumference. Myrrh's branches are covered with strong thorns and sparse leaves. The inconspicuous flower panicles produce an olivelike fruit that is bitter to the taste, and which gave the tree its name, "murr," meaning bitter in Arabic (Fischer-Rizzi, 1996).

Historical and Current Usage

Myrrh and frankincense seem almost inseparable in their history and use, as they have repeatedly been seen throughout different cultures as complimentary in their properties. In line with this, frankincense is often thought of as providing male energy and myrrh the female. Myrrh's earthy, warm, spicy balsamic fragrance is the yin (female quality) to compliment frankincense's lighter, spicy citrus balsamic scent that symbolizes the yang (male quality). Myrrh is a dark, dirty-looking resin that has no aroma unless it is smoldered, or unless the essential oils are extracted. Myrrh is often used in perfumery and aromatherapy. In perfumes it is used to lend a spicy base and an oriental character. As a flavor, it produces a biting-burning taste.

Legendarily, in Egypt the falcon god Horus created myrrh, and people who partook of this fragrance were promised to escape death and "become part of the eternal life of the gods." When Tutankhamen's tomb was opened the aroma of myrrh was still present. Myrrh was used not only in the embalming process but also as a varnish, a cement, and for making personal ornaments. The word *enbalm* is derived from the Latin *in balsamum,* meaning to preserve in balsam. The association of myrrh to women and feminine eroticism was inseparable in Egyptian love poems, and it was also used for medicine, magic, worship, and as a calming influence for troubled minds of both the sick and healthy. Egyptians called myrrh "bal," which meant "to drive out the insanity." Myrrh and frankincense were considered the most valuable objects one could own, for as long as the Egyptian empire existed (Fischer-Rizzi, 1996).

Myrrh never became as popular as frankincense in the Roman Empire, but it did become much more expensive, and therefore it was used as a status symbol. Myrrh was seen as a luxury even for the dead, as it was burned during cremations. In the classical times of the Roman and Greek gods, myrrh was believed to also have originated through a story of love. Myrrh was once a woman who had fallen in love with her father (Classen et al., 1994). Both frankincense and myrrh were present in Greek mythology, and as all aromatic plants, was thought to originate from the gods (Fischer-Rizzi, 1996).

The sacred Jewish anointing oils specified in the Old Testament contained myrrh as the main ingredient. Hebrew women were also prescribed specific cleansing rituals that involved the use of fragrant substances. One of these was the generous use of myrrh. The early use of myrrh was also either of the pure resin or a processed form of the bark (fresh bark boiled and pressed) called stakte. Supposedly, stakte was more costly, and was the form of myrrh that was brought to baby Jesus upon his birth (Langenheim, 2004; Fischer-Rizzi, 1996).

Frankincense and myrrh were mentioned the same number of times in the bible, but frankincense became preferred for divine worship, although both were present in many rituals. Frankincense was associated with Christ's divinity, whereas myrrh was associated with his persecution and death. Jesus accepted myrrh handed to him as gifts both at his birth and his death. One of the customs before a man was executed was to give him myrrh wine, because it acted as an anesthesia (Langenheim, 2004; Fischer-Rizzi, 1996).

Myrrh was synonymous for Indian frankincense (also Indian Bdellium, or Guggulu, Guggal, and Guggu in Hindi). In the ancient Arab world it was used in a similar manner to frankincense—people burned it in the home and at altars for sacred worship and offerings. In Ayurveda, common myrrh is able to increase Pitta (a type of dosha or energy in the body that is fiery in nature). It is also thought to be soothing for stomach tension, nerves, and rheumatism, and to be able to strengthen the uterus, ease sciatica, and for treatment of psoriasis. In India it is often combined with benzoin resin (Fischer-Rizzi, 1996).

Myrrh has long traditional and current uses beyond incense use including as a dye; the charcoal is used for cleaning teeth, strengthening the gums, and for wound healing; and a preparation of the bark has been used to treat skin disease (Quezada, 2003). The resins from the various species of myrrh have been particularly used for medicinal purposes in Indian, Arabian, and African cultures. In India the indigenous species *(C. wightii)* is well known for its use in medicine. Its guggulsterones have been well studied, and the resin, called guggulipid is well known to be hypolipidemic, anti-inflammatory, and antioxidant, and is often used as an adjuvunct to treating high cholesterol. Guggulsterone has been confirmed to lower cholesterol in clinical studies, and is also a potent antioxidant (Wang et al., 2004). Guggulipid is also used for treating arthritis, rheumatism, and other vascular conditions (Soehartono and Newton, 2002). *C. myrrha* is used by Middle Easterners for numerous reasons, including as an antimicrobial agent, stimulant, mouthwash, for the stomach, and for cancer. The myrrh resin from this species has been proven to be an antioxidant and antitumor agent that also is able to stimulate the thyroid and reduce prostaglandins. In preclinical studies, it performed well as a standard anticancer drug, cyclophosphamide, in its antitumor activity. Moreover, a couple of its sesquiterpenes have been shown to have potent analgesic activity. *M. guidottii* contains T-cadinol, which has smooth-muscle relaxing properties (Langenheim, 2004). Myrrh has several similar medicinal qualities as frankincense because they share some of the same terpenoids in their resin (Langenheim, 2004).

Known Chemical Constituents

Guggulsterone is known to be an active medicinal component of myrrh, which is able to lower cholesterol, be lipid lowering, be a cardioprotectant, and is a good antioxidant (Wang et al., 2004; Singh et al., 1993). Sesquiterpene lactones in (Commiphora) myrrh are thought to be responsible for its known activity of slowing tumor growth, and also for its antihyperglycemic activity (Zhu et al., 2003). Myrrh essential oils are known to have an antihelminthic activity (Kakrani and Kalyani, 1984). The resin of several myrrh species has been found to be anti-inflammatory (Duwiejua et al., 1993). The gum resin of myrrh has been found to consist of alpha pinene, myrcene, unidentified eugenol, cadinene, unidentified, geraniol. methyl heptanone, d-alpha-phellandrene, d-limonene, (+-) bornyl acetate, 1,8-cineol, unidentified, (+-) linalool, methyl chavicol, and alpha-terpineol (Saxena and Sharma, 1998). The essential oil has an LD50 of 705 mg/kg intraperitoneal (ip) and 1,669 mg/kg orally (Fischer-Rizzi, 1996; Bagi et al., 1985).

SANDALWOOD: SWEET SENSUOUSNESS

Scientific names: *Santalum album* L. (others exist in trade including *S. austrocaledonicum, S. latifolium, S. spicatum, S. yasi, Amyris balsamifera, Eremophila mitchelli, Fusanus acuminatus [Santalum acuminatum]); Vetiveria zizanioides; Adenanthera pavonina; Pterocarpus santalinus*

Common names: Indian Sandalwood; Byakudan (Japanese); Australian sandalwood; Sandalwood fan; Red sandalwood (used for dyeing).

Plant family: Santalaceae

Origin: *S. album* is indigenous to and widely cultivated in India, but China and other countries are now cultivating sandalwood. Sandalwood used to come primarily from the Mysore forests, but today it is probably coming from Tamil Nadu, as the Mysore forests have been overharvested. Sandalwood production was found to be decreasing in the early 1990s, and since then efforts have been underway to restore production through better management of sandalwood plantations (Rai and Sarma, 1990).

See Photos G.22, G.23, and G.24 in the color photo gallery.

Sandalwood is usually sold in the form of raw wood chips, splinters, powder, or forms (beads or figures). The sandalwood tree does not produce a good quality incense product until the essential oil content of the wood develops fully, taking often more than twenty years. The true sandalwood tree is grown in the eastern Indian regions of Mysore and Karnataka, and it is said that the tree has some relationship with the soil that develops the fragrance in these regions, and if planted in other areas the oil will not develop the same high-quality scent. Australian species of *Santalum* are also popular as "Australian sandalwood," and are used for incense and are distilled for fragrance and medicines (Quezada, 2003). "Sandalwood" from the West Indies, Venezuela, and Jamaica are mostly *Amyris balsamifera,* which is an unrelated plant.

Sandalwood oils are of various qualities, and many have been found not to meet the internationally recognized standard for sandalwood oil of having 90 percent santalol content (Howes et al., 2004).

Description of Plant

The sandalwood tree *(S. album)* is partially parasitic, able to photosynthesize, but also sends roots down to nearby trees to aid in its nutrient absorption. It can grow up to thirty-three feet, with a diameter of seven feet, and it is evergreen with soft-looking branches. It takes at least fifteen to twenty years before trees produce sufficient essential oil content, and the tree does not reach full maturity until sixty to eighty years (Fischer-Rizzi, 1996).

Historical and Current Usage

Sandalwood is an excellent incense for those who are first learning to use incense and identify their scents. It is an ancient incense with a woody fragrance that is warm and sweet and can be smelled before it is even burned. The wood is often used to make prayer beads and spiritual icons for its fragrant and spiritual qualities. Finely pulverized sandalwood is also used as a fragrant body powder after bathing by women in India. Its fragrance is considered to be calming and relaxing for those who are undergoing stress, and it is also known to alleviate headaches (Fischer-Rizzi, 1996).

Indian sandalwood is grown for its many uses in India. The timber is used for making chests and for burning at Buddhist funerals. The ground wood is used as a body powder and for cosmetics. It is also used as an incense, for making fragrances, in medicine, and it is one of the pigments used in caste marks (Quezada, 2003). In Hindu tradition, sandalwood is important in almost every phase of life. During a cremation of a wealthy Hindu, chunks of sandalwood are added to the fire to support the person's journey into the next phase of life (Fischer-Rizzi, 1996).

Although it is primarily thought of as connected to Indian traditions, sandalwood was an important incense ingredient for the kyphi mixtures in ancient Egypt, one of the most popular incense and fragrance blends of those times. Sandalwood is also highly revered in Ayurvedic and Tibetan medicine for its medicinal properties. Sandalwood is seen as possessing a strongly vital energy, and in Ayurveda it is considered bitter, cooling, relaxing, and contracting. It has been used to treat respiratory tract and kidney infections, skin irritations (as a paste), and for headaches. In living spaces it is considered to be antibacterial as well, and is blended into clarified butter to be burned over coal (Fischer-Rizzi, 1996).

In Japan, although it is not used in *Koh-do* ceremonies, sandalwood is available and frequently used in the home. It is available in square chunks, and a shaving may be placed on a mica plate for burning (Fischer-Rizzi, 1996).

Santalol, the main component in sandalwood oil, has been found have anti–skin cancer activity (Dwivedi et al., 2003). Sandalwood oil has also been found to have an anti-candida activity (Hammer et al., 1998). Research has also found that the sesquiterpenes present in sandalwood and released as the incense smoke, may increase the oxygen levels in the brain by 28 percent, which undoubtedly may produce other benefits in the body, such as an increase in the activity of the hypothalamus—and its subsequent effect on emotions, learning, and attitude—and may improve immune function, hormone balance, and energy levels (Williams, 2004).

Known Chemical Constituents

Sandalwood contains sequiterpenes, sesquiterpenols, and sesquiterpenals, santalic and teresantalic acid, aldehyde, pterocarpin and hyrocarbons, isovaleric aldehyde, santene, and santenone. Sandalwood oil is usually standardized to 90 percent santalol content, one of the essential oils present in sandalwood that is thought to be the cause of its characteristic fragrance. Santalol has a z-alpha and a z-beta form. Twelve known compounds of the sandalwood oil *(Santalum album)* are: tricyclokasantalal, alpha-santalene, trans-alpha-bergamotene, beta-santalene (S and E), alpha-curcumene, alpha-santalol, beta-santalol (S and E), nuciferol, alpha-santalal, and beta-santalal (Yu et al., 1988).

SWEETGRASS: A BRAID TO ATTRACT GOOD SPIRITS

Scientific name: *Hierochloe odorata* (L.) Wahlenb. (similar to *Anthoxanthum*).

Common names: holy grass; buffalo grass; vanilla grass; zebrovka.

Plant family: Poaceae.

Origin: Sweetgrass grows naturally in the prairie areas of North America and Canada, and in Europe (Fischer-Rizzi, 1996; Pignatti, 1979). Sweetgrass is a long-bladed grass that is often braided together and dried. It may also be used in small cuts, as some may be cut or shaved off of the braid in order to place on charcoal.

See Photos G.25 and G.26 in the color photo gallery.

Description of Plant

This grass loves moist soils, and may be found in the wild in the prairie or it may be cultivated. The base of the grass may have a reddish hue to it, but overall the blade looks green. It is a perennial grass that grows in clumps. Sweetgrass's native habitat is in the American prairies that extend up into Canada, and it is also found in Europe.

Historical and Current Usage

The Latin (scientific) name for sweetgrass, *Hierochloe,* comes from the Greek word *Hieros* which means sacred, and *chloe,* meaning grass. Sweetgrass is a good name for describing its scent, because when it is burned it emits a sweet, grasslike fragrance that is somewhat similar to sweet woodruff. This is the characteristic scent of coumarins. It is a pleasing scent when burned, but has very little until scent until it is smoldered.

Sweetgrass is historically used as a "medicine" or ceremony plant by Native Americans, especially the Lakota (Sioux), and also as a basket weaving component (Galluzzi and Kimmerer, 2003). Sweetgrass is a very important plant in Native American culture, and it is used for prayer and during smudging. It may be used to bless or purify certain people, places, or objects, and it is also given for welcome and parting gifts. It is often used in the sweat lodge traditionally (*inipi* ceremony), along with cedar, to bless the first seven stones ("grandfathers").

Sweetgrass is used to attract good spirits or positive energy to a ceremony or space, or is used as a blessing. Whereas white sage may be used to first cleanse a space of negative energies or spirits, sweetgrass is often used afterward to attract positive spirits. Sweetgrass is also used to scent clothes (Quezada, 2003).

According to Chief Phil Crazybull, a medicine man of the Lakota:

> Sweetgrass is harvested from the water. It is a form of acknowledging to the spirits that we honor life from water. We honor the plant that came from the water and all the animal spirits. We forget that what feeds us and clothes us has to do with the animal world, as well as the plant world which also feeds us and clothes us. And so when we use the sweetgrass we are asking spirits of these here nations to come and help us (the animal and plant world). We can't do things alone, we have to rely on that which is more powerful than we are. Because we say that even (the) bear is more powerful than we are, the ant is more powerful than we are. Because they can stay out in a storm in thirty-two degrees below zero, and if there was a flood we would drown

and they wouldn't. And so they are more powerful than we are, and so we have to always ask for their help so that we can use the sweetgrass to acknowledge those entities that are stronger than we are, that water, those animals and plant nations that live under the ground. So we always ask for their help.

Sweetgrass calls them to help us. We can never do anything to please anything, or anyone, so we do it to acknowledge them and to call them. It can be done as often as you could because its something that is hardly ever done anymore. My grandma used to do it every day. We had a iron stove that we used to put cedar and sage and sweetgrass, and other plants, and we would put them on there, and their aroma would take off all over the house. But that was back then, today we do it all separately, we used to have it all together in one bag and boom—grab a handful and put it on there! (Crazybull, personal communication, February 2004)

Sweetgrass is used by a number of Native American tribes for various uses, including as a medicine (for both humans and animals) by the Blackfoot, Cheyenne, Flathead, Kiowa, Menominee, and Plains Indians, for its use as a fiber for such things as in baskets or mats by the Iroquois, Kiowa, Menominee, and Micmac. Many of these same tribes also use sweetgrass ceremonially, as well, and for purification, for the sweet smell, for smoking, for purifying Sundancers, for protection, as an insecticide, and as a hair wash (Okugawa et al., 1996).

Sweetgrass is also used in traditional medicines for colds and fevers, as a painkiller, and as an insect repellant. Extracts of sweetgrass have also been found to be potent free-radical scavengers (antioxidants) (Pukalskas et al., 2002).

Known Chemical Constituents

Coumarins are responsible for the characteristic scent of sweetgrass. 5,8-dihydroxybenzopyranone and 5-hydroxy-8-O-beta-D-glucopyranosyl-benzopyranone, constituents of sweetgrass, have been identified as possessing significant antioxidant activity (Pukalskas et al., 2002; Bandoniene et al., 2000).

VETIVER: A COOL RELAXING SCENT

Scientific name: *Vetiveria zizaniodes.*
Common name: Vetiver.
Plant family: Gramineae.
Origin: Vetiver is native to India, and is now introduced and culti-
vated in many rural tropical areas of the world.
See Photo G.27 in the color photo gallery.

Description of Plant

Vetiver is in the same family as the sweetgrasses that are also used
in incense. It is a robust, grasslike plant with strong roots that spread
deeply and laterally under the soil surface and help to protect land for
erosion.

Historical and Current Usage

Even in small amounts, vetiver produces a strong earthy and sweet
scent, which many consider to be heavy and erotic. In aromatherapy,
vetiver oil is popular for relieving stress, anxiety, tension, and insomnia. The root is used in dried and often pulverized form. Essential oil
from vetiver root is also very common in aromatherapy and incense
products. Its oil is viscous and is brownish, amber, or olive in color,
with a deep smoky and earthy sweet scent. Vetiver may be used as the
dried root or root powder for an incense, or it may be added into incense sticks in the form of essential oil.

Vetiver has many traditional ethnobotanical uses, including as a
carminative, stimulant, and diaphoretic. Vetiver essential oil has been
found to posses sedative activity; to exhibit antifungal activity when
tested against *Aspergillus niger, Aspergillus flavus, Fusarium
oxysporum,* and *Penicillium* spp (Gangrade et al., 1991); to have antibacterial activity against *Staphylococcus aureus* and *Streptococcus
pyogens* (Gangrade et al., 1990); and to have nematocidal activity
(Nakamura et al., 1990).

Vetiver is used in Ayurveda for its many recognized activities including, cooling, calming, soothing, and alterative activities. It is
used in numerous conditions in Ayurveda, including for vomiting,
thirst, bladder infections and conditions, burning sensations, flu, fever, insomnia, hysteria, and asthma. In India, because it is a native

plant, it has a long tradition of use by many of the different tribes in India for such ailments as burns, bites, stings, rheumatism, and fever. In some regions a cooling drinking water is made from soaking the roots in it, and hanging dried vetiver roots is common for imparting fragrance. One of these uses is as blind, woven from the root mass, that is hung during the hot summer days. The blind is soaked in water several times daily, and as the hot air passes through it, it becomes refreshing as a bittersweet aroma is dispersed (Chomchalow, 2001).

Vetiver is used as both a medicinal and aromatic plant by people throughout Asia and India, including Nepal, Thailand, and Indonesia. In Indonesia, Vetiver is used for treating body odor by drinking a cup of the boiled root in water daily. Vetiver is also used to treat rheumatism, for pest control, and also as an aromatic fan on hot days. In Sri Lanka, Vetiver has similar cooling and urinary tract uses, and it is also used as an incense for its sweet scent (Chomchalow, 2001). In Senegal, Vetiver is used as a calming agent and for emotional stress. It is also used as an aphrodisiac, water purifier, and antibacterial. Older women wear belts made of Vetiver to increase their good scent and attract men (Chomchalow, 2001). In Pakistan, Vetiver is used medicinally for several conditions, including for heart palpitation and fainting, fever, inflammation, and irritable stomach. Vetiver as an incense is also used to treat headaches (Chomchalow, 2001).

Known Chemical Constituents

The main constituents of the essential oil of Vetiver are vetiverol, vetivone, khusimone, khusitone, terpenes (e.g., vetivenes), and sesquiterpenoids. The main polysaccharides present in vetiver grass are hemicelluloses (approximately 38 percent) and cellulose (approximately 27 percent). The protein content is about 5 percent, lignin 10 percent, and ash 3 percent (mainly silica) (Methacanon et al., 2003).

WHITE SAGE: BIG MEDICINE

Scientific name: *Salvia apiana.*
Common name: California sage; white sage.
Plant family: Lamiaceae.

Origin: North America (coastal from northern Baja California to northern Santa Barbara county); usually wild-harvested but sometimes cultivated.

See Photo G.28 in the color photo gallery.

Description of Plant

White sage lives up to its name as it displays rather large white/gray leaves and stems and pure white flowers. It grows to about five feet when in ideal conditions, but can be limited to a much smaller, scrubby plant in drier conditions, with leaves growing in rosettes similar to cabbages. Once one is familiar with white sage, it is difficult to confuse with any other, as its lush white leaves and scent is distinctive. Brushing a hand along a branch and rubbing its leaves gives off a strong scent that is definitely sagelike, but also a little sweet.

Other plant species may be sold, erroneously or commonly called "white sage," including *Artemisia californica* (California sage). *Salvia apiana* may be cultivated, and many nurseries are beginning to carry the plant for growing in areas without much frost.

Sometimes when sage is dried improperly it may become moldy. Check sage before burning to assure that it is not moldy, otherwise it will effect its scent.

Historical and Current Usage

In North America this plant is commonly used in Native American ceremony, as well by countless "new agers" and other Westerners who may use it in their home for purification, to create a more spiritual effect, or for prayer and meditation. In Native American ceremony it is used commonly before and sometimes inside the sweat lodge for purification or clearing the air. White sage is thought to chase away bad or evil spirits and be "clearing" in this manner. The leaves are used either loose or tied together (with stems) in a bundle to form a "smudge stick." This is a favored incense (usually called "medicine" or "smudge") by Native Americans. Other plants are sometimes used as "white sage," but this one is the only true sage (*Salvia* spp.).

White sage is most commonly found in new-age book/crystal stores or health food stores for sale as a "smudge stick." A bundle of sage is usually tied together by a string and dried, sometimes along with other plants inside the bundle. Other sage species and nonsage (not Salvia) genera are sold as "white sage." The American Indian Movement (AIM) contends that the selling of white sage, or other sacred medicines, is disrespectful, and has actively asked many stores not to carry it for sale (Vernon Bellecourt, personal communication, May 5, 2005).

Another common perception of sage is that it supports mental clarity and wisdom—thus it is the cause for the word "sage" to describe or name a person of wisdom. Other types of sage have been used since ancient times in many cultures around the world for similar reasons. Sage tea is thought to protect the body and spirit, and it is also known to reduce perspiration (Fischer-Rizzi, 1996).

In Native American spirituality, it is used as a smudge in a similar manner to cedar in honoring and purifying oneself and others. It is for guidance and as a protector, and can help to call the spirits and get rid of bad spirits and bad energy in a space. It can help also to purify and protect the home, and guide someone to speak the truth. According to Chief Phil Crazybull:

> It is the spirit of the plant that comes with the smudging. It is not only your spirit, but also the ancestors of who you are, [who] are brought into the realm of this here smudging that creates an aura of all that has been before and all that is coming this way. It helps you in guiding someone to feel and to understand that there is a communication between you that is going to benefit mankind. (Crazybull, personal communication, February 2004)

He added that most sage is white because it is the color that relates to the ancestors, just as ghosts are often depicted as white, so are all ancestors white. So white sage has that tradition of use of relating to the ancestors. It is one of the most commonly used smudging plants in the Native American traditions. According to Chief Phil Crazybull:

> We use sage in our Sun Dances in our hair, our crowns, our bracelets, ankles, and wrists. And we use sage in our vision quests to lay down, and to equalize in our house the powers of our ancestors, and to protect them. And so sage has many, many uses besides being smudged—we use it in our pipe bags, we use it to help heal people, to help cleanse people, to help protect people. And so sage has been a very powerful element of our

whole way of life. It is something that is so practically used that we forget what its purpose is. (Crazybull, personal communication, February 2004)

White sage is also sometimes consumed as a food. Its seeds may be consumed raw or cooked, and it may be mixed with cereals (such as oats or wheat) and also toasted as a powder and dried. The seeds are also used as a spice, and they may be soaked overnight to be used as a drink for water or fruit juice. White sage is also used as a traditional medicine to be consumed internally. Sage tea is made from the leaves, and is good for coughs, colds, and as a blood tonic. The incense is also used for cleaning the air of a room as a fumigation after someone with a contagious disease has inhabited it. The seeds are also used as eye cleaners (Okugawa et al., 1996).

Other traditional Native American uses include as a hair shampoo, and as a dye and straightener (leaves crushed in water). The leaves may be crushed and made into a poultice to be used on the body and under the armpits as a deodorant (Okugawa et al., 1996).

Known Chemical Constituents

The leaves contain up to 4 percent volatile oils, including camphor and eucalyptol, ursolic acids, oleanolic acids, alpha-amyrin, abietane diterpenes 16-hydroxy-carnosic acid (making from 1 to 2 percent the dry weight), and carnosic acid (Moore, 1993). An antibacterial and antifungal compound has been found in *Salvia apiana,* called 16-hydroxycarnosic acid (Dentali and Hoffmann, 1992). A number of abietane diterpenes have been reported from the roots of white sage (Gonzalez et al., 1992).

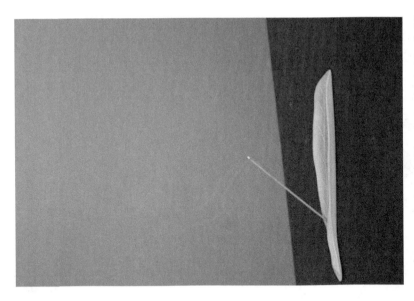

PHOTO G.2. A leaf-shaped incense stick holder holding burning incense.

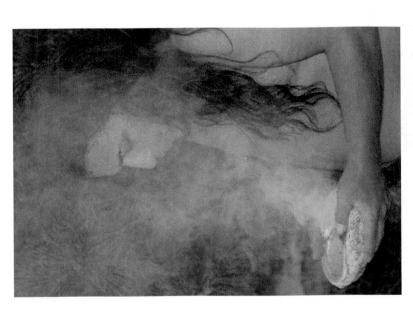

PHOTO G.1. Native American Nicholas Sanchez smudging himself with white sage.

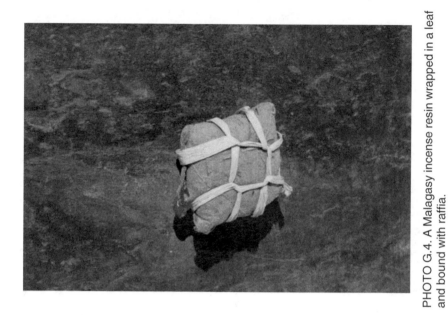

PHOTO G.4. A Malagasy incense resin wrapped in a leaf and bound with raffia.

PHOTO G.3. A natural incense mixture composed of resins, seeds, leaves, and bark.

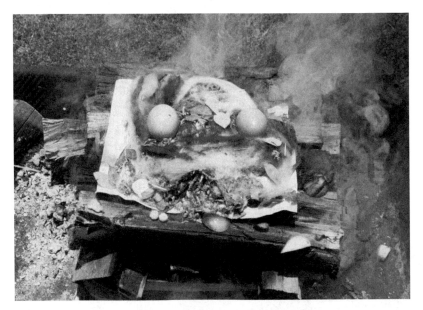

PHOTO G.5. A Bolivian offering (containing incense resins) to be burned on a fire in a house blessing ceremony in La Paz, Bolivia. Prepared by Rufino Paxi.

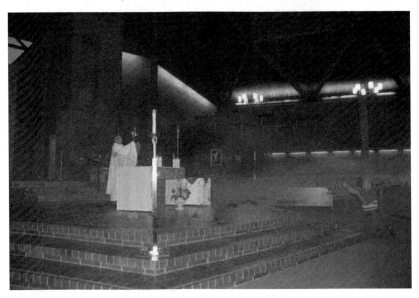

PHOTO G.6. Incense offering during Benediction in a Catholic church.

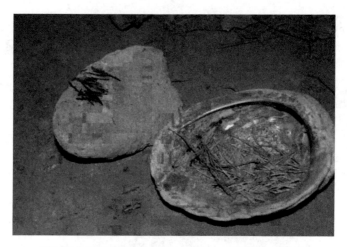

PHOTO G.7. Cedar smoldering in an abalone shell.

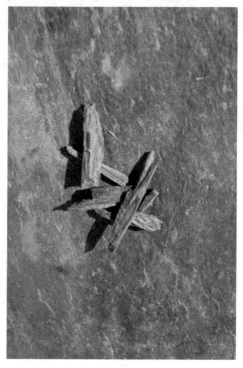

PHOTO G.8. Chips of agarwood.

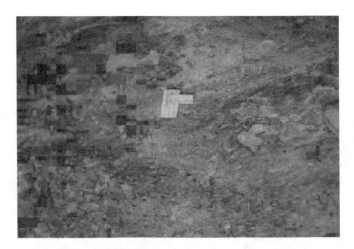

PHOTO G.9. Chips of agarwood as found in *Koh-do*.

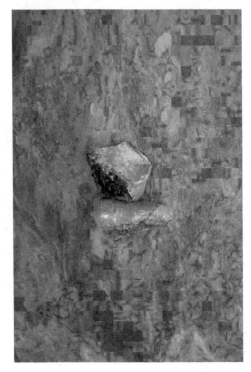

PHOTO G.10. Balsam of Tolu.

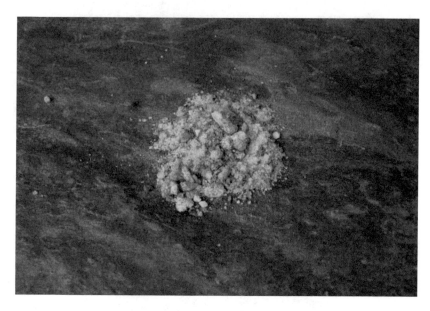

PHOTO G.11. Benzoin of Sumatra.

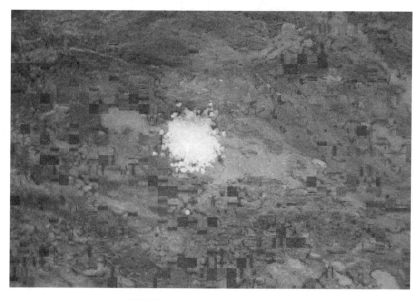

PHOTO G.12. Borneol camphor.

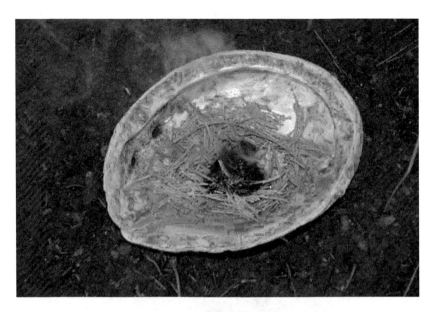

PHOTO G.13. Cedar in an abalone shell.

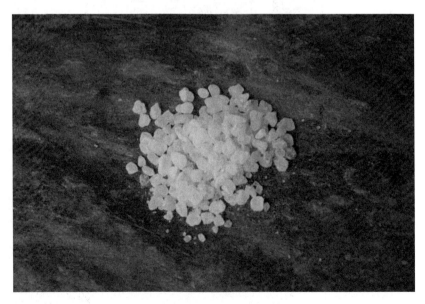

PHOTO G.14. White copal.

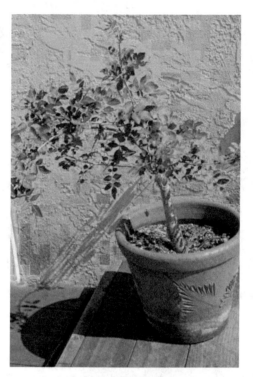

PHOTO G.15. A small sapling of a copal-producing species.

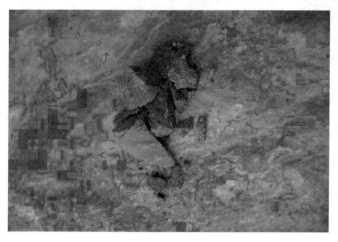

PHOTO G.16. Dragon's blood resin.

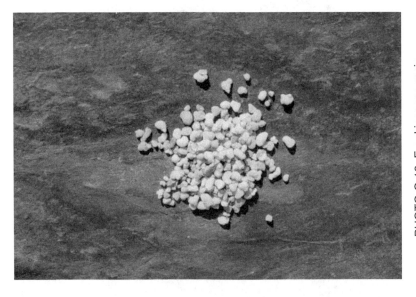

PHOTO G.18. Frankincense resin.

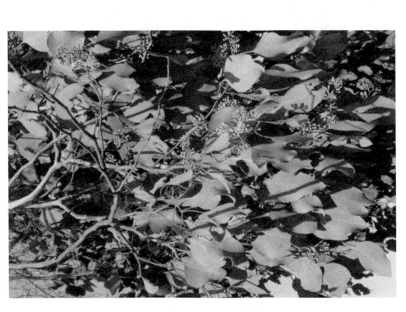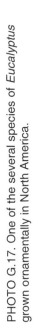

PHOTO G.17. One of the several species of *Eucalyptus* grown ornamentally in North America.

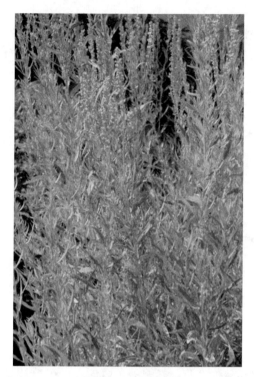

PHOTO G.19. A California native form of mugwort.

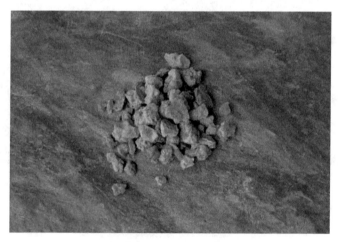

PHOTO G.20. Myrrh resin.

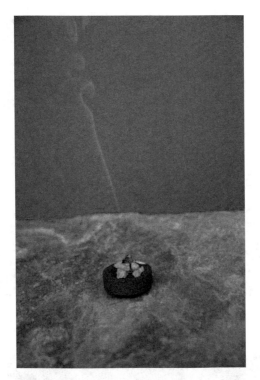

PHOTO G.21. Myrrh smoldering on charcoal.

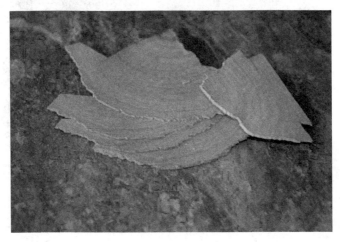

PHOTO G.22. Sandalwood shavings to be used as incense.

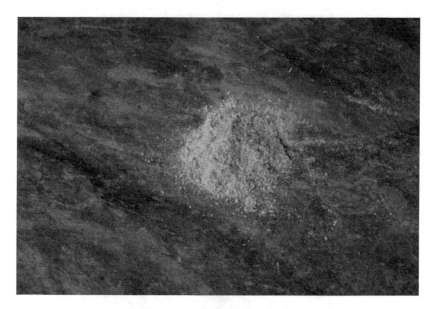

PHOTO G.23. Sandalwood powder to be used as incense.

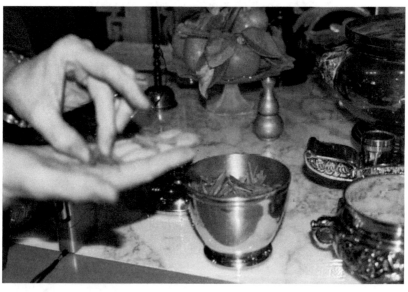

PHOTO G.24. Chipped sandalwood for use as incense at a Buddhist temple.

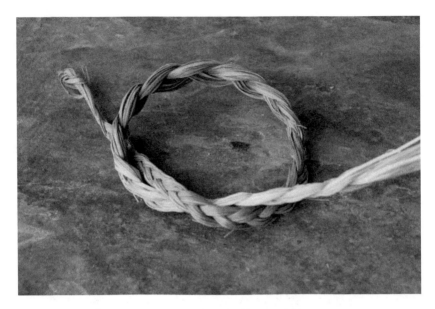

PHOTO G.25. Sweetgrass braid.

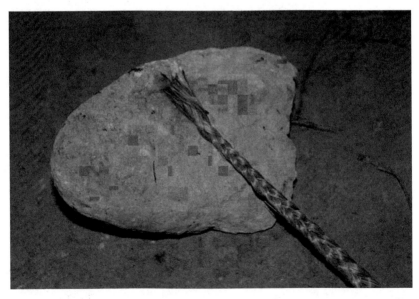

PHOTO G.26. Sweetgrass braid smoldering on a hot rock.

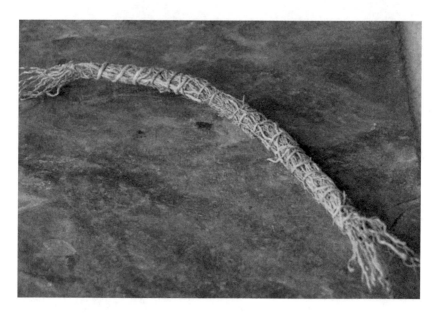

PHOTO G.27. Vetiver.

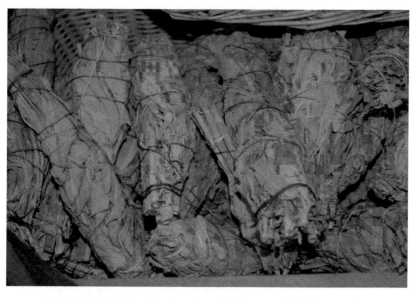

PHOTO G.28. Smudge bundles of white sage *(Salvia apiana).*

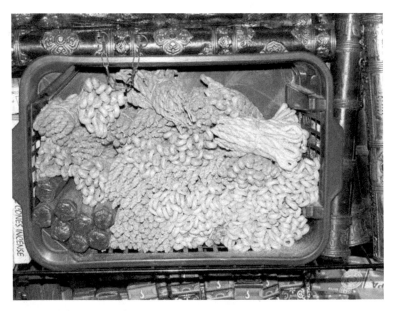

PHOTO G.29. Braided incense ropes.

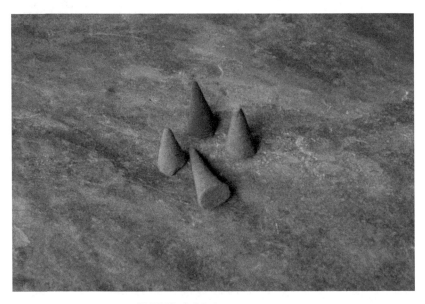

PHOTO G.30. Incense cones.

Chapter 5

Bringing It Home

Now that we have seen the pervasiveness of incense around the world, and how it is found in many rituals and cultures, and now that we have also gotten to know some of the plants, how do we bring this all home? This chapter covers some of the basic knowledge of making incense, offers a description of the incense forms you may encounter, and a discusses some of the symbolism of incense and its various components.

MAKING INCENSE

You may decide that making incense is not for you, and, at least in the beginning, you will want to buy forms of incense that are already on the market. This is a good strategy, but I caution you to try to find incense that is a pure as possible—free of synthetic oils or substances. Since this is a difficult task, I have included a resource list in Appendix A that may help to guide you or get you started. However, many simple forms of incense can be made that you can start with if you decide you want a more personal connection with your incense.

One of the easiest ways that incense is made is by bundling together leafy herbs, similar to a smudge stick. White sage or another fragrant leafy incense burning plant (such as mugwort) may be picked (the leafy stems) and then bundled together and dried. You may hang the bundle upside down, or even just dry single stems and pick off the leaves for use singly as incense. The more aromatic kinds of leafy incense will burn without any other help. Just ignite one end, and blow out (or fan out) the flame. The leaves should smolder continuously, and the ignited portion will work its way to the base of the bundle eventually, as the fragrant smoke is released.

Another way to make incense is to put together blends of single ingredients, and then to burn them on lighted charcoal or coals. Many incense blends exist that you may research, or you may find out on your own what you like the best. To do this you need to invest in either charcoal tablets or in some other form of incense-burning material, or an incense stove.

You may also make incense cones or sticks (or other forms) by putting together four basic materials into an incense mixture that can be formed. This is not meant to be a guide for doing it yourself, only a simplified outline of the process, and more can be learned by purchasing other incense books. The four basic materials are as follows:

1. *The scent.* The first step is to decide what kind of aromatic substance you would like to give the mixture its characteristic odor or qualities. Herbs, spices, and resins may all be used. Chapter 4 gives more information on single forms of incense.

2. *The base or chemical burning agent.* The next step is to choose the base for helping the mixture to burn evenly and easily. Some bases have a scent, and some have no scent whatsoever. Bases can be chosen to interact with the aromatic substances in the incense and can balance the aroma of the main scented herbs/resins that are too strong by themselves. A base can make the aromatic portion of the incense milder, less bitter, and less pungent in order to make an even-burning and good scent. Popular bases include mixtures of wood powders, sandalwood, vetiver, evergreen needles, and willow. In either case, the base should be ground to a fine powder. Talc is sometimes added to the base in order to lengthen the burning time. Saltpeter, also called potassium nitrate (sometime also sodium nitrate is used), is one of the drawbacks of using a blended incense cone or stick, as nearly all contain saltpeter in order to help them burn. Saltpeter should not be added directly as a powder; it needs to be dissolved in a liquid (see number 4) so that it can be more evenly distributed in the incense so as not to cause flare-ups, or burnouts. Natural alternatives to saltpeter are available, but rare. I have never experienced this myself, but others explain that if the exact right mixture of resins and woods are put together in making a combustible incense formula, sometimes it will burn without saltpeter.

3. *Bonding gum/agent.* In order to pull together the aromatic portion and the base, a bonding gum is needed. Typical gums that are useful for this purpose are agar agar, ghatti gum, guar gum, gum Arabic, locust bean gum, karaya, tragacanth, sodium alginate, and xanthan gum.
4. *Liquid.* In order to turn the bonding agent into a glue, a form of liquid, such as water, is needed. However, a number of substances can be used, including wine, brandy, rose water, and olive oil.

Generally the proportion of these four materials are twenty parts aromatic substance, four parts base, and one part bonding agent, although this may be altered depending on the strength of aromatic substances used, or if pure essential oils are being used. All the substances are mixed together in a powdered form (except for saltpeter), and then liquid is added in order to bond the substances together with the glue that is formed. The mixture then can be made into cones or cylinders and set to dry. Incense sticks are made using various processes, from hand rolling, to extruding from a mold, to hand dipping, and they all produce a form of stick incense that is pure and easy to use.

FORMS OF INCENSE

A number of different forms of incense are commonly used. Certain religions, such as Catholicism, may only use one form, and others, such as Buddhism, may use a number of forms. Some forms are more familiar, such as stick incense or joss sticks, and others may be completely foreign to you, such as a braided sweetgrass in Native American tradition. You may want to experiment with a few until you find the one that you would be most comfortable with, or which stimulates you the most.

A word of caution about buying Native American incense at stores or shops: The American Indian Movement (AIM) has issued warnings or declarations to stores that carry Native American forms of incense (such as smudge sticks). They consider these substances to be sacred medicines, and do not condone the buying or selling of them (Vernon Bellecourt, personal communication, May 5, 2005).

Loose Leaf/Bark/Wood or Resin Incense

Much of the discussion in this book has focused on the use of raw incenses, such as the sweet resins, wood, loose leaf, or flowers that are either directly used as incense or are mixed into special blends and used for making other incense forms such as cones, sticks, spirals, etc. This is one of the most ancient and pure forms of incense use, and is common to almost all traditions that use incense (see Photos G.3 in the color photo gallery and Photo 5.1).

Smudge Sticks

Smudge sticks, or smudge bundles as they are also called, are a common form of incense use among the Native Americans (see Photo 5.2). Generally it is a type of white sage (leafy branches) that is bound together by string and then dried. Once the smudge stick is dried, the

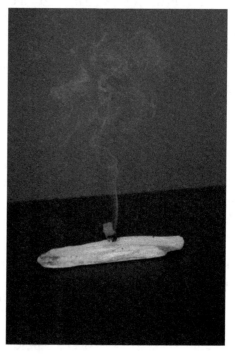

PHOTO 5.1. Palo Santo: A type of smudge (incense) from Latin America that can be lit directly or used over hot rocks or coal.

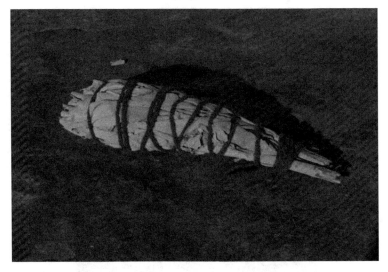

PHOTO 5.2. Stems of California white sage *(Salvia apiana)* that are bound together in a smudge stick, dried, and then used as an incense (by lighting one end).

smudge stick may be used as is (as long as the string is made of a natural flammable material, such as cotton), or the string may be taken off, since a tightly bound smudge stick will stay together. The smudge stick may be initially difficult to light if it is bound tightly together, but once lit it will smolder and produce a copious amount of white smoke. The smudge stick may be held at one end, and then smoke may be fanned onto objects, persons, or throughout areas.

Braided Sweetgrass and Other Braided Incense Forms

Sweetgrass is another Native American incense that is often used in ceremony and sometimes available at bookstores or shops having to do with spirituality (see Photo 5.3). The sweetgrass is a type of long grass that grows in the plains region of the United States, and when used for incense, it is braided when still in the ground, then tied at the top and the bottom and later cut. The entire braid is then carried to ceremony, or placed on the altar, and when used it may be either lit at one end, placed upon hot and glowing rocks to smolder, or shavings of the grass may be placed on charcoal or glowing coals or rocks.

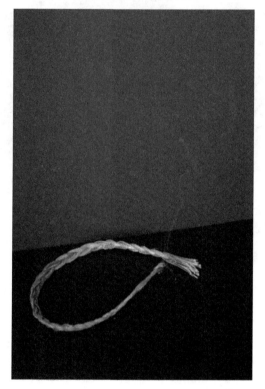

PHOTO 5.3. Sweetgrass: A commonly used Native American medicine and type of smudge (incense).

Other braided forms of incense exist in different areas of the world, such as in China, where braided incense ropes are used as an inferior type of incense (see Photo G.29 in the color photo gallery).

Chipped Incense (Shokoh)

This is a mixture of five, seven, or ten ingredients that is used primarily on Buddhist altars. The main ingredients are usually jinkoh, sandalwood, ambergris, cloves, and ginger, and mixtures may vary in quality, as many poor quality mixtures with adulterated ingredients are on the market. A pinch of the chipped incense is placed on a bowl of hot ashes, or less commonly onto horizontally burning joss sticks (laying side by side) (Morita, 1992).

Incense Balls with Blends (Nerikoh)

This is a time-consuming process in which incense materials are hand ground and then blended with honey or plum meat into balls and placed in a ceramic jar to be buried for at least three years. Since many variables affect how the scent of *nerikoh* will turn out, each ball is said to have its own uniqueness, and manufacturers that produce them guard the recipes as secrets (Morita, 1992).

Joss Sticks (Senkoh)

Originally, joss sticks were in the form of a blended incense ball on top of a bamboo stick, making it appear as a lollipop, but today joss sticks are commonly found in a stick form without the bamboo (see Photo 2.3 in Chapter 2). Joss sticks originated before the time of Buddha in India, and only after the Buddha's death did they become associated with Buddhist ritual. Not only do joss sticks function as a form of incense, but they also are used to measure time, as the incense burns at a constant rate (Morita, 1992).

Incense sticks were made in a manufacturing process that included extrusion, a process similar to the making of noodles, and from those early times the process has changed little today. In ancient China, wood dust would be combined with the bark of elm root and thinned with water. To this, fragranced powders would be added, including clove, camphor, and/or cypress. These would be thinned in Chinese wine, and made into a paste. This would all be placed into a pump that extruded the mixture into noodlelike sticks, which where cut at the ritual lengths (usually between fifteen to eighteen centimeters). These sticks were then tightly packed into bundles or nineteen, thirty-seven, sixty-one, or ninety-one—the numbers of sticks that would fit into a cylindrical bundle of various sizes (Bedini, 1994).

A regular fourteen-centimeter-long stick burns for about twenty-five minutes, an eighteen-centimeter-long stick for about fifty minutes to one hour, and a seventy-three-centimeter-long stick, which is more common in temples, will burn for about eight hours. Several ingredients (between seven and fifteen ingredients) may be blended together in a joss stick, including *jinkoh*, bark, cloves, amber, and the Japanese Judas tree *(Cercidiphyllum japonicum)*. The latter ingredient has a only a very mild fragrance, and it is used to bind all the ingredients together (Morita, 1992).

Incense Cones with Blends (Ensuikoh)

Incense cones are similar to the joss-stick incense in their manu-facturing process; however, instead of being pushed through holes to form the spaghetti-like sticks, the blended incense is pressed into cone-shaped molds (see Photo G.30 in the color photo gallery). The cones became popular in the 1960s when exporting them was much easier than exporting the sticks due to the breakage of the long sticks (Morita, 1992).

Sachets (Nioi-Bukuro)

Sachets are technically not incense because they are not burned; however, they are included here because they contain many of the same ingredients and are clean to use for those with an intolerance to smoke. Essentially, the same incense ingredients would be placed not into a dough to make the incense form but into a bag or cloth, and then placed into drawers or clothing, or hung around the neck or in the room. The sachets were worn or hung not only to emit their pleasant fragrance (which they did for about a year) but also to repel ill-fortune (Morita, 1992).

SOME INCENSE MATERIALS AND SYMBOLS

Incense use is both tangible and elusive, and its use throughout the world has much symbolism attached to it. This symbolism may be found in the very vessels that are used to burn or hold incense, or they may be found in the many aspects or utensils used in the ritual of burning and dispersing incense smoke.

Incense Vessels and Censers

Many different kinds of incense-burning vessels exist, and range from the very simple bowl, to elaborately shaped containers that are made to swing from the hand, to electric stoves. One of the most familiar images among Westerners is the type of censer that is used in the Catholic Church, usually a bronze or shiny metal, and shaped like an urn, with a lid with holes (see Photo 1.1 in Chapter 1 and Photo 5.4). This is usually suspended by three long chains and held at the

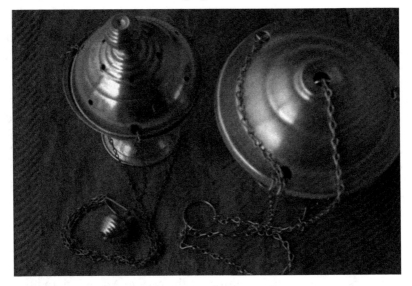

PHOTO 5.4. Censers.

top where the chains come together. Inside this type of censer might be placed a disk of the quick-light charcoal, and then resins of frankincense placed on top. These may be swung while walking down the aisle of a church, as is the job of a thurifer, or they may be hung. This type of censer was developed in the ninth century; before then priests used just a basic open vessel that was carried through the church. Italian and Spanish Gothic-styled incense censers were particularly elaborate, and were often depicted in cathedrals as being swung by angels.

Any container will suffice, however, especially if it is one that is fireproof, such as a ceramic bowl. Salt, sand, or ash may then be used to cover the bottom of the bowl and prevent it from burning the surface below it. Charcoal tablets may then be placed on the sand, or incense sticks may be stuck in the sand and allowed to smolder until it reaches the base. Even more simple is the use of a rock that has been heated in a campfire, or charcoal. Sweet resins or other raw incense materials may be placed directly on top of these and smoldered. However, if you are a person that wants to deeply explore the art of incense burning, an endless array of incense burning vessels and stoves are available throughout the world.

The "hill censer," invented in China, was one of the first censers to be manufactured especially for the burning of incense. The hill censer was made either of pottery or bronze, and was similar to a goblet, with a separate lid that was hill shaped, with two rows of waves surrounding it. The hill censer then inspired many other forms, including using the heads of beasts and birds in the design, and the another type of censer called the *ting*. The *ting* was similar to a small cauldron, and was supported by three or four legs. Many of the manufactured censers took shapes of cauldrons and forms of old times, but the hill censer was the first from which the manufacture of censers begun. The *pei chung hsian lu* is another special Asian censer that is used for the perfuming of clothes (Bedini, 1994).

Temple Utensils

A number of utensils may be used in the burning of incense, depending on the ritual and tradition. In the Native American tradition, antlers or even pitchforks and shovels may be used to move or place the hot rocks or coal that the incense or medicine plants are placed on in order to smolder. In the Japanese art of *Koh-do,* and in some Buddhist traditions, a number of utensils may be used, each with their prescribed way and time to use them, such as ash presses, feather-tipped brushes, chopsticks, spoons, tweezers, electric wood-chip heaters, mortars and pestles, storage boxes, and wafting feathers (Hyams, 2004).

Incense-Stick Holder

Even more familiar than censers are the many shapes and forms used as incense-stick holders (see Photo G.2 in the color photo gallery). A never-ending supply of forms can be made into incense stick holders, with many that come to be holders accidentally. Some of my favorite kinds of holders are those that never meant to be, such as potted houseplants. I have one houseplant (a ficus tree) that has so many broken ends of bamboo skewers and unburned joss sticks in the soil that I can barely find room to add one more incense stick. The strange part is that the plant seems to like the attention. Perhaps there is something after all to the idea of plants responding in growth and vitality to our attention, such as when people sing to them.

Feathers

Feathers have a common association with incense around the world, and much symbolism ties birds and fragrant plant smoke together. According to the Native American tradition, birds and feathers carry sacred medicine just as plants do. When a feather is prayed with, it is thought to bring those prayers to the Creator, and it may impart healing powers of the bird's medicine. The bald eagle was considered among the most sacred of the birds by the Native Americans long before it became the symbol for the United States. One reason for this is because the eagle is the bird that flies the highest in the sky, and thus the closest to the creator. During incense use then, feathers may be waved to waft the incense smoke toward people or objects, and they may also be prayed upon. Fanning the charcoal may also help to bring oxygen to burn the incense.

In ritual, incense smoke is often dispersed into the air with a feather. Someone told me (or maybe I read) that the feather symbolized the "breath of life." If incense can represent the scent of gods, or (as in some Buddhist practice) the direct teachings of Buddha, how fitting that it is dispersed by "the breath of life." Feathers are most mortal in their physical form, but in function, how immortal and divine.

Charcoal

Charcoal used to burn incense is available in specialty/spirituality stores (see Photo 5.5). It is important not to use the charcoal briquettes used for barbecues, but to use special incense charcoals, or the larger temple quick-lighting tablets that are usually available in a roll of ten. They are specially designed for incense use in censers, are available in many different sizes, and are easy to light. One of the drawbacks, however, is that they give off a small charcoal odor (especially the larger ones in the form of disks), and so if you are using very high quality incense woods or small amounts of delicate incense, the charcoal tablets may be both too hot and impart too much odor for effective use.

When lighting a charcoal tablet it is best to hold it with tweezers, or some utensil that protects your fingers from scalding. The charcoal tablet may take several seconds to light when you are holding a flame to it, and it may also spark and crackle a little as you are doing this.

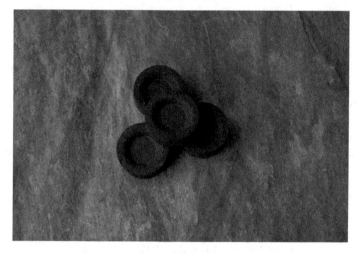

PHOTO 5.5. Commonly found charcoal disks.

When burning a large amount of heavy resins on a charcoal tablet it is best to wait for the tablet to burn a little first because the resins may smother the flame on a newly lighted tablet.

Other types of charcoal are available that are more natural and may impart less odor. A type of natural burning agent called makko powder can be used in place of potassium nitrate. Japanese charcoal has no odor, is more elegant, but also is more expensive. A charcoal made of coconut husks that is said to be free of toxins is used by some Indian manufacturers. In Brazil, "vegetable charcoal" tablets (that look like marshmallows) made of fragrant woods that burn slowly are available in various Candomblé and "macumba" shops (Hyams, 2004).

Electric Burner/Incense Stove

Although electric burners are available for burning incense, they will deprive the experience of the use of fire, which is an integral part of the symbolism and ritual. However, several electric burners are available that are made in Japan of fine porcelain, with a fire stone or small metal bowl for burning the incense. Another type of electric incense burner made in areas were incense is a part of daily life, such as Dubai, can fit into a vehicle's cigarette lighter. The advantage of these burners is that they burn clean and slowly, so that the full fragrance of delicate woods can be appreciated (Hyams, 2004).

Fire and Smoke

Fire and smoke are integral parts of the incense experience, so they should be regarded as sacred and not be feared. So often we don't allow the use of fire or burning of candles in our houses for fear of the houses burning down, but if fire and smoke are carefully used they may be safely enjoyed. Make sure that the surface the incense receptacle is set on is fireproof, and that the incense is never left unattended in the house when in use.

Smoke is also an important part of incense, for without it there would be no incense! Not long ago in history smoke was a part of daily lives, and has been for about as long as we have been on this planet. In many cultures smoke symbolized the bounty and hearth of a healthy home. However, recently, with the prolific addiction of our society to cigarette smoking, smoke has gained a bad reputation and is thought of as a harbinger of the toxic additive chemicals that are manufactured by the cigarette companies, not to mention its being a by-product of industrial pollution. Adding insult to this is the use of synthetic materials in candles and incense, which cause many irritations and allergic reactions. Moreover, the poisoning of our air with automobile and industrial poisons and smog has brought our collective conscious to the point that "fresh air" is air with no fragrance, no smoke, and no man-made chemicals.

We have forgotten that fresh air normally comes with the slight fragrance of resinous trees from the mountain, or the slight, sweet, earthy odor of the composting forest floor. Step out of your car when you arrive in the mountains and take a whiff. Most likely you will notice the delicate, camphoraceous, piney scent of evergreens, or the scent of cold, melting snow, or that reassuring fragrance of campfire smoke.

Although we can reach out to incense and learn its craft, forms, and symbolism, once we look up we can realize that incense has been with us all along. It is present in the simple pleasures of life. It is the smell of a campfire, the fragrance of the evergreens, and the scent of a flower. And with these associations it has the powerful ability to transport us and connect us to what really is the most important.

Chapter 6

Nature's Divinity Awaits

I don't feel like writing a poem,
Instead, I will light the incense-burning vessel
Filled with myrrh, jasmine and frankincense,
And the poem will grow in my heart
Like flowers in my garden

According to a student of Hafis (fifteenth century AD)
(Fischer-Rizzi, 1996)

Let My Prayer be set fourth before thee as incense (Psalm 141:2)

(Hyams, 2004)

Do you ever feel trapped in the concrete jungle that surrounds you, or in the confines of your own life? Have you learned to run faster and faster, and have forgotten to "take time out to smell the roses"? It's an old saying with a wise meaning, and smelling the roses may just be a necessity of a healthy life. Using incense can help us to regain connection to the natural world, which many of us have deadened ourselves to, as many people done in many types of spirituality and religion throughout time and across the world. There are many different reasons to use incense, but somehow the specific reason that we may have in our conscious mind doesn't really matter. Once you inhale the natural, sweet smell, you will *feel* why it is you want to use incense.

As the "way of incense" in the ancient Japanese culture was just as important as the tea ceremony, a list of the Ten Virtues of Incense was summarized by a Zen priest in the sixteenth century:

1. It awakens your senses to a higher level.
2. It purifies mind and body.
3. It removes uncleanliness.
4. It keeps one alert.
5. It can be a companion in the midst of solitude.
6. In the midst of busy affairs, it brings a moment of peace.
7. When it is plentiful, one never tires of it.
8. When there is little, still one is satisfied.
9. Age does not change its efficacy.
10. Used every day, it does no harm. (Morita, 1992)

As you start sampling different kinds of incenses and blends you might consider keeping an incense journal to note how each incense affects or inspires you, and what kind of mood it evokes. You may follow the example of the Japanese, and start writing poetry that is inspired by the incense, and describe the seasons and elements of nature the incense releases.

You may also want to create an altar to house your incense and any of your sacred objects, and to act as a space to focus your daily meditation and/or prayer. An altar may be suited to your particular religion, or have objects on it that are important and sacred to you (see Photo 6.1). It does not have to be in a room that is dedicated only to spiritual practice, although if you have this it is excellent for meditation, martial arts, etc. Your altar, rather, can be placed in the corner of your bedroom, living room, or any other room in your house that you have a special affinity for and find most suited for quiet contemplation. Find a place in your house that can act as a special focus place for your spirituality, faith, and/or quiet reflection. It can be a personal altar or a family altar. Things that are typically found on altars are images of deities, candles, incense, pictures of loved ones that you want watched over, flowers, or sacred herbs. You may want to smudge or purify the air in the room with sage, as is common in the Native American tradition.

DIFFERENT USES OF INCENSE

Although incense use shares many common elements around the globe, a diversity of different purposes for using incense exists. In

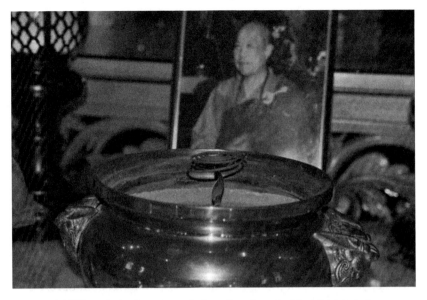

PHOTO 6.1. An incense spiral on the altar at a Buddhist temple.

practice, we may be using incense for several different purposes at once. Following is a discussion of many areas of incense use.

For the Unification of Mind, Body, and Spirit

Incense can affect the mind, body, and spirit, and is an excellent remedy to unify those parts of you that you feel are out of alignment. Incense can affect the mind by either focusing the mind, or relaxing it and calming it from many of the busy thoughts that run around daily through our heads. It can both take us out of the present and transport us to vivid memories of the past, and it can also deepen our awareness for the present and help us to live more fully in that moment. Essences have also been called spirits, as nothing is as otherworldly yet tangible as is incense. It is our go-between in realities, and used for this reason throughout the world. It is both of heaven and of earth, and because of this it can accompany our spirits and help ease spiritual transition. Incense affects us so deeply it is able to change us, all the way down to the molecular level. Most of all it is able to stimulate our own body to heal itself in the way our bodies already know best.

For the Aroma: To Create Your Own Paradise

Our concept of paradise normally contains the natural aromas of the good, sweet plants of a lush environment that drench the air around us. They are sweet and balmy and accompany our minds in our peaceful bliss. Just as the Garden of Eden was thought to be located at the origin of many of our most ubiquitous incenses—such as frankincense and myrrh—it too was described to contain fragrant odors (Atchley, 1909).

Incense use may go no further for you than this—just as many people are attracted to the idea of using scented candles and potpourris, incense can act as a daily ritual in creating your own home paradise. Or perhaps you may bring this paradise with you to work, and help your co-workers in an unseen way. Imagine how much nicer people might act if they were less stressed out and were soothed by the environment around them. Incense, if used properly, can have this effect. I have a friend who is a therapist, and he would burn copal before and sometimes during sessions to help his clients to open up and feel at ease.

If your co-workers or family members are sensitive to smoke, you may try using the incense when they are not around, so that only the scent lingers in the air and they are not bothered by the smoke. Also, choosing which incense to burn is important as some are more smoky than others. Try smaller quantities of a sweet resin, such as copal, frankincense, or myrrh, and compare this to more smoky mixtures containing cedar or sage.

A Buddhist monk of the Chan tradition, Heng Sure, explains how the essential idea of incense is to adorn this world to make it better:

> What I do is hold a stick of incense up between the eyebrows and contemplate that while I am offering this single piece of incense, at the same time, if my mind is pure, then I can with my contemplation send it out so that it permeates throughout the universe. Buddhism talks about how this is not the only world operating at this moment, so that if your mind is pure you can actually connect with other worlds. This one offering then becomes bigger than the one offering. The purpose is that incense can purify the nose so that the perceptions are enhanced, and it is a way of adorning the world. If you can adorn this world, you

can move into a better world. (Heng Sure, personal communication, December 2, 2003)

To Perfume the Clothes, Hair, and Body

Incense has been used in several cultures throughout time as a perfume, in many ways one could consider it the most ancient of perfumes. One of the best ways to use incense as a perfume is to hold whatever item you would like fragranced above an incense vessel (but not so close that it burns the item), and let the smoke envelop it and permeate it with its fragrance. This ritual has been performed for clothes, linens, bedclothes, and even hair, and is still popular in many parts of the world, such as Arabia. Specially designed enclosed censers with holes in the top, which will prevent hair or clothes from getting burned, may be used for this purpose. In Japan, women used to lie with their hair draped over a special censer while their hair was fragranced. Such rituals do not leave the clothes or hair smoky smelling, as one might imagine, and if good quality incense is used it will create a lasting perfume of sweet aroma that others will notice and enjoy.

If you have a good towel rack, you do not need special censers in order to perfume clothes or linens. You might hang the items to be censed on this, and place the censer below. Or if you have a walk-in closet, or a closet that is closed off, a censer may be placed on the floor (or some other safe place) and left to smolder. All sorts of incense substances are good for perfuming, although the sweet-smelling ones are particularly recommended for scenting hair and clothes, such as the sweet resins sandalwood, copal, and aloeswood.

The ancient Hebrews also used to enjoy such perfuming rituals, especially after the priests abolished the law disallowing people to use incense. Women had specific cleansing rituals, including the use of incense as a perfume for their clothing and blankets, and King David was said to cense his royal clothing in order to tempt the daughters of neighboring kings (Fischer-Rizzi, 1996). I recently scented my clothing, and throughout the day felt that people were noticing the scent. Several that hugged me remarked that I smelled good, but more often they said I looked good, and it seemed they were unaware of what made me look more attractive that day (since I did not dress or do anything unusual besides scent my clothes). Perhaps it was only my attitude that made the difference as the sweet, spicy scent was with me throughout the day in a subtle way, and it did make me feel special. Either way, I suggest for you to do your own experiment and find out for yourself.

Meditation

Probably one of the most frequent uses of incense in the world, considering the number of Asian and Indian Buddhists, is for use during meditation. However, meditation is becoming a useful technique for non-Buddhists living in industrialized countries who need a way to relax and be more present in their lives. Stress is eating at our health and meditation has been proven to calm the mind as well as the body, bringing many health benefits to those that practice meditation. Incense can play a role as a helpful aid in centering and grounding the mind and getting it ready for meditation. During meditation incense is a calming presence, helping to reduce some of the nervous chattiness present in the mind, and it may help aid the soul in spiritual transition.

According to Heng Sure:

> Buddhist meditation doesn't necessarily have any object in mind, the idea is that you are not responding to thoughts that arise. Yet it is not trancelike. You need clarity—you are more alert and awake then before you meditate. Most people don't have any idea how murky their minds are until they sit and meditate. It is like opening a closet and all this stuff falls out. So the mind is the same way once you sit you begin to clean it up.
>
> If you contemplate, that has a focus. You may want to contemplate compassion. You go from your own experience to something more universal. The other way is to just observe what comes up. You may have thoughts such as, "when is this meditation session going to end?" You notice yourself getting impatient, and notice and contemplate who is watching, and then let it go. You just react to what ever arises—you observe it and let it go. Another kind of meditation is called "cessation meditation." In this kind of meditation, as thoughts come up you stop them and just sweep them away. (Heng Sure, personal communication, December 2, 2003)

A number of incense blends and types that are common to Buddhist practice make excellent meditation companions. However, you may find your own scent that has a calming and grounding effect on you, or you may prefer one that opens your conscience to more spiritual energies, uplifting your own energy to those higher planes.

Finding Your Vision and Your Dream

In many cultures throughout the world, dreams are important for helping people understand something about themselves, and for helping them to find purpose and direction in life. The Tibetan Buddhist practice includes a special form of yoga: dream yoga. Through this dream-work practice it is thought that if one is able to master awakening in dreamtime, then one would also be able to awaken to the illusion of our daylight existence. This is in relation to the teaching in mystical Tibetan sacred texts, such as the *Wheel of Luminosity* and the *Tibetan Book of the Dead,* which is that our waking existence is just a daytime dream. In some cultures, such as the Native American Lakota, certain people in the society are adept dreamers, and they are valued for this gift of dreaming that they have been given as a tool for helping people and for giving direction to the whole tribe. Some people might call the dreams prophecies. These dreams or visions are not just the every-night kind that are forgotten, they are "big dreams," ones that you feel and see so intensely that they stay with you. The Native Americans believe that these dreams are here to teach us, if we pay attention. According to Chief Phil Crazybull:

> A lot of dreams are created by ones own ambition to be something or somebody. But spiritual dreams are those that are connected to ones career and ones ability to make something happen so that it honors them as a human being. The dreams show them how to honor themselves and the creator at the same time. (Crazybull, personal communication, February 2004)

He explained that these kinds of dreams may not be complex, and they are often very simple because that is who we are—"simple human beings." For example, if you were a singer you might have had a dream that you were standing by the water and whole crowds of people came to hear your sing. This simple dream, explained Chief Crazybull, indicates that you should offer water to the spirit world,

and before going to sing, drink water. It is almost common sense because people often need the water to clear their throat before they
sing, anyway. He added:

> These dreams are basically very simple, because that is who we
> are; we are simple human beings. In some ways we are very
> complicated, but in some ways very simple. But to honor spiri-
> tuality in the Lakota way is very simple. It is not something that
> we have to go through a half an hour ritual or something like
> that, it is just very exact and to the point. Because that is how life
> is, we say, one moment you might be alive and the next you
> might be dead. And so it is simple, quick and to the point. (Chief
> Phil Crazybull, personal communication, February 2004)

Certain kinds of incense, such as cedar, have been used to help
people connect with their visions and dreams. Finding your purpose
in life so that you may not only help yourself, but help others, can be
done through dreaming and finding visions. Everybody is different in
their natural ability to dream and to attract vision. But even for those
of us for whom dreaming does not come easily, certain activities and
methods can be used to help us strengthen our dreaming and to help
us find vision in our lives.

Cedar may be used for this purpose not only in ceremonies, such as
the sacred Native American ceremonies of the Sun Dance, the Sweat
Lodge *(Inipi),* and Vision Quest *(Hamblecha),* but it can be burned in
the home to help us develop our dreams. Cedar is also good for helping us overcome nightmares (Chief Phil Crazybull, personal communication, February 2004).

While sitting in meditation or working in the garden, try burning
cedar over some charcoal, and place it in an area where the smoke can
create an atmosphere around you. Learning to attract vision can be a
difficult or long spiritual process, but for some it is easy, and visions
just come. However, take caution that your are not just imagining
what you want to see. Surrender to what comes, and then try to understand the relevance for your life. As Chief Crazybull explains:

> So maybe sometime you use the cedar and you see a horse, and
> you think, *what is the meaning of the horse?* It has something to
> do with you, nothing to do with what is out there but what is to
> do with you. And that can be essential to helping another per-

son, and that is what a lot of times we use cedar in the ceremony to do, [to find an answer to] What is your purpose? A lot of times people ask me this: "What is my purpose?" "What is my purpose in life?" [I tell them] "Well, have you ever used cedar, have you ever dreamed of the things you want to do?" People have always said, "reach for the stars," "reach for your dream." Well, what is your dream, what is your purpose? We say that one purpose is that you help one human being in your lifetime find their path and find themselves, so they can honor the creator, so they can honor their life. So they can do something to help their own self and their own families, and that is the beginning. To begin by helping one person. (Chief Phil Crazybull, personal communication, February 2004)

Connectedness

You may have heard the saying that we all just want to belong. At the root of this feeling is the true connection that we all crave to feel alive and part of the unrestrained wilderness that reflects the deep mysteries of the universe. Some people know this feeling as a desire to know God, others think of it as a longing for family and community, but what it all has in common is the feeling of connectedness.

As Heng Sure the Buddhist monk explains,

> I think brokenness, separatedness, is probably the main source of suffering in the world. Certainly it is harder to harm someone to whom you see your relationship. Being "separated from" is fundamentally not true in the Buddhist context, and when someone wakes up they see how related we are, how interdependent we are. Lack of awakening—the opposite of that—is feeling that the *things I do don't matter,* that *I got away with something.* For example, seeing the earth as a commodity is unawakened, whereas seeing the earth as a community is closer to the truth. Meteorology connects us, the markets connect us, entertainment markets connect us, ecology connects us. When these professionals using scientific methodologies look at the world they see it this way, but when it comes down to people they break it into tribes.
>
> One of the best parts of our human nature is the wish to look beyond what comes to us, to wake up. The great sages and prophets of all traditions see further, and why are we inspired to

gaze through their eyes? Because it is bigger. What we see through their eyes is the bigger connection, the bigger pattern. Anybody who has laid on his or her back and looked up at the sky immediately has to ask, "Where is the limit?" Our culture is failing because of the separating we do. We drive our car into carports, and we push a button and the door goes down, and we go into a big house where we rattle around. In Barcelona, the culture is in no danger of falling apart. You go out at ten thirty at night and people are all out on the sidewalk relating.

People ask me all the time, "How do I meditate?" One of the first questions I ask in return is, "When was the last time you called your mother?" In order to become a person you need to repay this filial kindness. Even if the relationship is not good, it needs to be a wholesome relationship. If you want your mind to be quiet and big, you need to connect with these roots from which the groundwater of humanity comes. You need to make the relationship with your mother at least connected. If it is painful, you need to at least own half of that pain. So heal it, and make it peaceful in your heart. One good way to do that is to say "thank you," and that is *connecting*. (Heng Sure, personal communication, December 2, 2003)

Incense can help us on our path to find the connection we desire. Whether we use it in religion and spirituality on our path to knowing God, during meditation, or just around the house during a quiet moment, it can have the powerful effect of triggering our ancient memories of what it means to be alive. Incense in its tangible, yet intangible state can also help us to understand the nature of the Great Mystery.

It is important to find that incense may trigger deep, good feelings in you. As it is also connected to certain ritual uses, such as in death and in certain religions, however, it may also trigger negative memories. Some people may have negative feelings toward incense if they were exposed to it at a funeral, or during negative religious experiences. As Harvest McCampbell (2002), author of *Sacred Smoke,* a book about Native American use of incense, wrote:

Grandmother took me to the woods. She showed me how everything is alive and full of Spirit . . . how everything communicated...[h]ow even I could become part of it all, could become full with the beauty of the world.

Our desire for a sense of connection is not a luxury—without it we become ill in the mind and body. The sense of connection brings with it health, and health brings life.

Many people are at ease with the idea of having connection to other people, and sometimes to animals, especially their own pets. However, many of us have lost our sense of connection with plant life. Not only do most of us not know the names of the common plants that surround us, but it is rare to find a person who really knows the qualities of a plant let alone its uses or function in an ecosystem. These are all things of common knowledge in more traditional cultures.

So how do we regain that connection to plants, and thus to nature? The answer is that it is quite simple, and does not require us to drop out of society and live in a teepee. Many approaches can be taken, and it all depends on what works best for you. Some people feel a deep connection just walking in the woods. If this is true for you, perhaps you could slow down and look a little closer at the plants you pass. Pick just one or two to start. What environments do they live in? Are there other plants you typically see growing with them? What does the soil look like? One can learn may aspects of a plant. You may choose a more unconventional approach, however, such as that suggested by Connie Grauds, a natural medicine pharmacist, and author of the book *Jungle Medicine.* She suggests trying to get to know the spirit of the plant itself. One approach is by picking a little piece of the plant, and going to a place, such as a warm grassy field, where you can lay down peacefully and shut your eyes. Take a whiff of the plant, shut your eyes, and let your mind daydream. According to Grauds, sensitive people may be surprised that they could find themselves on a journey with that plant, maybe even talking to that plant's spirit. Getting to know plants in this way can help people open themselves up to a new consciousness, and bring them to that magical connection they may have had with nature in their youth.

Another simple technique is through incense. A similar process whereby a person either daydreams or meditates with the scent of incense in the air can help open the mind and create a connection with the divinity in nature.

Sacrifice

The thought of incense use and sacrifice conjures images in many people's minds of ancient animal sacrificial offerings. However, the idea of sacrifice occurs in many kinds of religions, and it usually is simply meant as a type of offering to the divine. As incense is often thought to appeal to the divine, it is often used in this way to attract God's attention or the attention of other spiritual energies (Atchley, 1909).

Another principal present in many kinds of spiritualities is suffering. By offering incense, or making a sacrifice of incense, we may suffer a little in the process, since we are giving something up (even if we enjoy the fragrance in the process). The idea of suffering in this sense can be easily grasped by people if a high monetary value is placed on the incense. Since we paid a large sum of money for the incense and then burned it in a spiritual offering, we may suffer a little due to that loss of money. Suffering is an integral part of life, but how we view it and deal with it differs. In the Hindu and Buddhist viewpoint, suffering is part of life, and only when one is enlightened can one rise above it completely. Meditation is one of the techniques that teaches our being how to rise above the suffering, and it brings us closer to enlightenment. In Christianity it is taught that this planet has inherited suffering due to man's sin. In Native American beliefs, suffering is part of life, and we must meet it as we take our place in the circle of life. Harvest McCampbell (2002) writes in her book *Sacred Smoke:*

> The mosquito suffers in the dragonfly's jaws so that there will always be dragonflies. The dragonfly suffers in the little bird's beak so there will always be little birds. The little bird suffers in the hawk's talons so there will always be hawks. I suffer the bite of the mosquito, so that there will always be dragonflies and little birds and hawks.

And so there are many ways to view suffering. As sacrifice may induce suffering, many ways to view the importance of sacrifice exist.

The making of an offering of incense, then, can be as a way of pleasing the divine, and it also may be a symbol of our sacrifice to God or spirits. Incense may also be burned as a way to thank God.

When Noah survived the flood and found his way on dry land again, he thanked God by burning myrrh and cedar (Hyams, 2004).

To Walk in Beauty (Purification and Cleansing)

According to Lakota spirituality, it is important to "walk in beauty" in life, and smudging is one of the first and basic steps to achieving this. Every morning the tip of a smudge bundle of white sage, or even a single loose dried sage leaf, can be smoldered and used to purify yourself. Not only is the earth polluted and contaminated by our actions and lifestyles, but according to Chief Crazybull, we also carry invisible contaminants around with us where ever we go that radiates to the world:

> As human beings we have an invisible aura about us that is good and bad that is creating pollutants to the earth. So in order to rectify that, we say that one needs to rectify that by using sage or sweetgrass or some of the elements that are created by the earth, so that when we walk out there we can walk in beauty. You can walk with the knowing that this invisible aura and pollutant that you carry is not hurting the earth, it is becoming one with the earth. (Chief Phil Crazybull, personal communication, February 2004)

According to Chief Crazybull, these contaminants are created partially by what we eat. In this sense the saying "you are what you eat" takes on a new relevance. All the processed and chemically altered foods that we eat are not only part of our bodies, but also part of a sort of invisible "aura" that surrounds us and emits to the rest of the world just how sick we are becoming (Chief Phil Crazybull, personal communication, February 2004).

Another source for these contaminants are our intentions. As Chief Crazybull explained, everything that goes through our minds begins with a process that is like a swelling in our bodies. When that swelling is caused by something that had ignited either happiness or anger within us, we emit that back to someone else in our aura. As Chief Crazybull distinctly pointed out, we not only emit to someone else, but to the land, the trees, and the animals, they can all sense it. Have you ever wondered how an animal is able to sense fear? Have you ever wondered why you are able to sense when someone is feeling down or angry? If we carry these emotions and intentions with us and emit them constantly, it is no wonder why we are a nation of fearful, confused, and angry people (Chief Phil Crazybull, personal communication, February 2004).

Smudging is seen not only as a way of purification, but as a way of protection and of guidance. Chief Crazybull tells of how it can guide us in making sure that our auras are not emitted to someone in an angry or competitive way, or to make people feel lesser than us, so that you feel equal with one another and at ease. Smudging is a daily ritual that anyone can do to help correct those bad intentions. As Chief Crazybull says:

> You always do it because you want to put the negative energy in balance with that which is good because we wake up with so many problems in our life—I gotta do this or I gotta do that. And we schedule so many things we have to, and we are so busy in life, so in order to put that back in balance you need to begin your day smudging so that the smudge is going to go with you where ever you go. (This is) so that you do not emit that kind of dominance with you that you carry, so that people can feel that you are not a threat, and there is something special about you that others don't really know, but in reality it is how you begin your day. (Chief Phil Crazybull, personal communication, February 2004)

So smudging is one of the ways to correct these imbalances within us, but other ways of doing this, of giving back to the land and saying "thank you," exist. Perhaps it can be through offering something, such as incense, or through a prayer. Chief Crazybull adds, "Among my people we just say one phrase: 'Mitakuye Oyasin' [meaning: All My Relations], and that is a prayer, a song, an announcement, a movement to get things moving, and we say that because everything is one, and we are one with everything" (Chief Phil Crazybull, personal communication, February 2004).

For Healings/Medicinal Incense

In many cultures, plants that are burned and inhaled are not called incense, but rather, medicines or smudges. In Native American cultures, plants are used this way often, and they are always called medicines, even if their outright intent is not some medical form of healing as we think of it in Western culture. In Tibet, a number of medicinal incense formulas have been used since ancient times.

The inhalation of or just prayer along with smoldering plants is considered a healing ritual in many cultures. The reasons for the incense's healing ability may be varied, including the direct inhalation of physiological healing compounds or mood-altering (and thus healing) compounds, as a sacrifice or symbol of our prayers to the gods, to clear the air of negative spirits or illness-causing presence, to attract healing spirits, and the list goes on. Essentially, incense is considered healing in almost every way it is used.

In Tibetan medicine, the central theory of what causes illness is a disturbed or pathological attitude of the human spirit, and these are caused by greed, hate, and ignorance. In this belief system, due to the mind/body nature of the cause of illness, incense burning mixtures have been created specifically for every type of psychosomatic cause of illness. The person undergoing treatment may then cover their head with a cloth, and lean over the incense bowl to inhale its smoke (Fischer-Rizzi, 1996).

In Ayurvedic medicine, the traditional medicine of India, since the Vedic times (1200-500 BC) incense has been administered in order to treat illness that is of a mind/body nature. This is in accord with the ancient beliefs of the sages that as humans we should aspire to be like flowers and emit only good words, good deeds, and good thoughts (Hyams, 2004).

The father of Western medicine, Hippocrates, thought that "the best way to health is to have an aromatic bath and scented massage every day." Just as incense is used in accompanying our prayers, so can it help us to heal.

Magic

Incense often has a negative association with magic and the occult. It is true that plants burned as incense are used for certain occult rituals and for magical incantations by "witches" of certain cultures. This association has occurred throughout centuries, and in the Western culture, perhaps it was never so prevalent as in the time of the alchemists. Books dating back to the time of Western Alchemy tradition can be found disclosing recipes for calling up the dead and their ghosts, and these recipes sometimes included known poisonous herbs that are well established hallucinogens. Common incenses, on the contrary, are known to be quite safe, and may provide us with a powerful journey to the divine without the use of psychedelics.

Another very common "magical" use of incense is for calling of plant spirits in shamanic traditions. Again, hallucinogenic plants are often used for this purpose, and some may be in the form of an incense or inhaled as smoke. According to the natural medicine pharmacist and student of shamanism, Connie Grauds, plant communication is subtle, and if we train our minds to hear their words we can hear them around us all the time. Perhaps the ability to "hear" the words of plants is not some magical ability that we gain through the use of psychedelics, shamans, or powers that we may or may not be born with; it is something we do every time we smell a flower!

For Creative Inspiration

As the word inspiration means to "breathe in," incense can and has been used for centuries as the artist's own divine muse. Incense both helps us to cultivate our "inner life" and helps us to birth that inner life in our creative endeavors. It is similar to a midwife who helps ease the transition of something that is often difficult, painful, and scary for artists. Even back in the classical times, the gods of the Greeks and Romans were so associated with scents that inhaling these scents were thought to have very strong effects on humans. The effect on these divine scents on humans was thought to be of an ecstatic and creative nature, able to inspire us divinely in our endeavors (Classen et al., 1994). As an artist may strive today to find divine inspiration from within themselves, incense smoldering in the artist studio may help to create the atmosphere and mind space for the artist. Incense may also be helpful for those of us who are searching to find our "true calling" in life, and spark that creative surge that brings out our true talents.

Even if you don't consider yourself a true artist, we all have the capacity to use the creative sides of ourselves. How would creativity enhance your work as a computer programmer, a mathematician, or a writer? A singer/songwriter, for example, may use incense during the songwriting process to inspire lyrics that come from the deep places within. They may also use an incense, such as frankincense, during the time of performance or singing, as frankincense has always been thought to enhance to quality and carrying of the voice in spaces. Perhaps incense may play a role in your daily life or work for inspiring your most divine work.

In Death and for the Soul to Make a Break from the Body

In funerals incense has often been used for various reasons. One reason is that in some cultures it was believed that a sweet scent was needed for the soul to be able to make a break from the body before it ascended to heaven or the spiritual dimension (Aftel, 2001).

One of the most renown uses of incense and spices for burial and funerals is that of the Egyptian mummy. The smoke of the incense was used to help send the souls of the departed to another world, and the next life. Not only were the fragrant resins and spices used as incense in these burials, but also in the process of embalming the body. The Romans were said to use lavender on funeral pyres among scented woods, and the Greeks burned Iris root as an offering to the goddess Isis, goddess of the rainbow and the messenger of the gods, so that she might escort the dead person on a rainbow to the "Land of Everlasting Peace."

The use of incense by some types of religions during burials, in fact, can be an unpleasant association for some people who have experienced this. However, I find that incense is a meaningful and comforting ritual performed in the memory of a departed friend. It is something meaningful that can be done in a time when there is not much else one can do. As Mandy Aftel says, "the pure of spirit aspire to become pure spirit—literally, to become scent," and the ethereal offering of incense can become both an offering to the memory of the departed, as well as a tangible sign of the deep mystery that now surrounds them (Aftel, 2001).

Improve Learning and Problem Solving

As discussed in Chapter 2, scents have a powerful link to memory, and scent is differentiated from the rest of the senses because of this direct link. This may help to explain why several clinical trials have been finding that scents can actually improve memory, learning, and problem solving. In these studies, certain aromas—including typical incense aromas such as lavender and sandalwood—were inhaled before performing certain tasks or during learning. The aromas were found not only to affect mood, but also to enhance certain learning and task-oriented skills. In other words, certain scents may be able to enhance our minds and moods so that our focus and alertness may be increased. It may also be possible that the scents were connected in our minds to the learning at hand, and just as certain scents can "magically" transport us to a vivid memory of a time or place, they may also be able to bring us back to the vividness of the learning experience. Much research still needs be done to understand more completely which scents affect what qualities of memory, learning, or task performance, but thus far the results have been encouraging.

So maybe the next time you are studying for a test, or typing a paper, an ambiance of incense smoldering in the background may help to bring you to the place of focus, relaxation, and creativity you need to focus and perform well at the task at hand.

To Mark a Rite of Passage and the Seasons

A common ritual use of incense throughout the world is to mark a rite of passage. For example, incense is used in many cultures to welcome a baby to the world: the Moroccans burn it on the day of a child's naming, the Sufis burn it to introduce a baby to life's deeper mysteries, and the blankets of North-African babies are scented with incense to protect them from evil spirits. Incense is also often used in weddings throughout the world. In Hindu weddings sandalwood and jasmine fill the air as the ceremony is performed (Hyams, 2004).

Another symbolic use of incense is for the marking and relation with the passing of seasons. In Japan, each season is marked by scents, and incense blends are specifically created to correspond to the season. The use of scents, the description of the natural world, and the description of seasons are integral parts of Japanese poetry. During the Vietnamese New Year, Tet, sandalwood and narcissus incense is burned on home altars to mark the new year and to give thanks and ask for blessings. A Chinese home may have a shrine to a kitchen god that is prayed to and offered incense, sweets, and candles, as it is believed that when the Chinese Lunar New Year is reached, the kitchen god travels to the Jade Emperor in heaven and reports on the behavior of the family that year (Hyams, 2004).

As the seasons of our lives pass, perhaps the best way to store these precious memories and times is in scents. The powerful ability that scent has to magically transport us to previous times may help us to live and appreciate life more fully. Imagine the happiest times of your life being marked by a particular sweet odor. Perhaps it is jasmine at your wedding. Now imagine being able to close your eyes, and inhale a whiff of jasmine, only to relive the experience again.

For Inducing Dreams and Sleep

Certain incenses have both the ability to enhance sleep, counteracting insomnia, and to induce dreams and visions. Those scents that are known to have a calming effect, such as lavender, sandalwood, and cinnamon, may be burned just before or during the bedtime (make sure it is in a fire-safe container). Many of these types of scents are both calming and also comforting, perhaps reminding us of happy and secure times. An example of this is cinnamon. The scent of cinnamon often has an association with holidays or baked goods, such as pies, which are associated with those safe and secure times in our lives when we are surrounded by loving family and friends.

Incense is also used in many cultures to induce dreaming and visions. This refers not only to the dreams of a good night's sleep, but to the more prophetic dreams that may be used to forecast the future or to give a glimpse of your inner consciousness. Examples of dream-inducing herbs are mugwort, white copal, and dream herb *(Calla zacatechichi)*. Dream-inducing herbs are also excellent aids for dream work and keeping a dream journal. They may help both the induction and the recall of such dreams. Scientific investigations at dream laboratories have found aromas to have a powerful effect on dreams (Trotter et al., 1988).

For Lovemaking

Incense often has an association with lovemaking and the more romantic times in our lives—if not those embarrassing times of making out and listening to loud music as teenagers. It is easy to get a glimpse of this association during a visit to a street-side incense stand in New York City. Large incense sticks that are sold separately or by the bunch are labeled as Black Love, Ecstasy, and Arabian Nights, among others. Most of these cheap incense sticks are made with synthetic fragrances (and not recommended by this book), however, it is clear what many people are trying to induce with such purchases. Just as the *Kama Sutra,* a book written on the "Instructions in the Art of Love" (see Chapter 3), describes fragrances as a key part of the love-making experience, incense has been used to induce a sensual mood and atmosphere for centuries. Cleopatra was said to be a master of this art, with her many tricks of using scented potions to entangle her lovers in desire (see Chapter 2).

Instead of buying the cheap incense sticks on the corner stand, however, I recommend finding incense that will allure, not aggravate, yours and your lover's senses. Sandalwood powder applied on the body or burned as incense is one easy and ancient fragrance of sensuality that is thought to elicit a divine union (Hyams, 2004).

Worship and Prayer

Hopefully this book has given at least a glimpse of the diversity of how incense is used in divine worship and prayer. From Islam to Christianity, incense has played an important and meaningful role in the history of most of the major world religions, and it is still a effervescent symbol of faith in many parts of the world. Included in the reasons for its use in divine worship and prayer are as the divine odor of the deities, a symbol of reverence and prayer, an offering to please the divine, as a demonifuge, and for purification or cleansing (Atchley, 1909).

The rituals involving incense use are even more diverse, yet are ever-present, in almost all the corners of the globe. From the use of smudge sticks in the Native American spiritual paths to cleanse a space, to the quiet meditation of monks before the image of Buddha, to the censer that is swung down the aisle during the procession of a Catholic Mass, many of these rituals have not been lost in history. Even common forms of incense, such as the incense sticks or joss sticks, have diverse uses through different cultures. Joss sticks may be broken, laid side by side, and used to burn chipped incense in a Buddhist meditation, whereas the Taiwanese may light both ends of a joss stick as "emergency incense" when they are in trouble (Hyams, 2004).

How you may use incense in worship and prayer is both a function of the religion or spirituality to which you belong and of your personal comfort and desire to bring it into your worship. Perhaps you will set up an altar at home for prayer and meditation. Perhaps you will enjoy the scent of frankincense only when you are attending a ceremony, such as during Catholic Mass, so that it remains special to you, or perhaps you care to bring it home to include in your daily prayers.

BECOMING MORE ALIVE

Many examples have been given of how incense may be used. We may deepen our meditations through the aid of incense, or we may be interested in incense for purely spiritual purposes, such as prayer or ritual. We may also be interested in incense for more banal daily activities, such as a pleasant scent around the house or for perfuming the clothes, hair, and body. Whatever your purpose, incense will gladly, silently accompany you.

With all the examples contained in the book of how incense may be used and why it may be used, along with the deep historical and present traditions, it is easy to see how incense is probably the most spiritual use of plants across the globe. Though few conversations have been initiated between religions about how this may unite us, and how it may connect us to the earth in an even more profound way, incense continues to be. It exists without much of our notice and it will continue to do so, whether or not we wake up to its presence.

However, should we care to take a new journey, and learn to see the world through the eyes of the divine, perhaps we can wake to not only the nature of incense, but to the true nature of ourselves. Why not light some incense, shut your eyes, and allow your sense of smell to magically transport you to memories of the past or paradises once lost. Let your sense of smell develop through the world of incense, so that you may now fully taste the richness of life. Let us deepen our

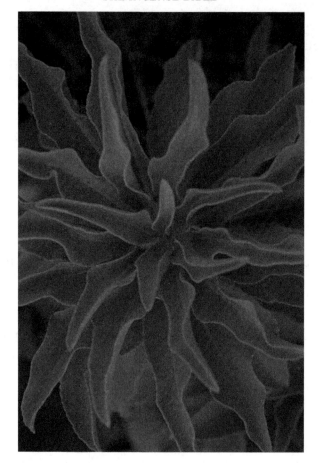

PHOTO 6.2. California White Sage: A highly regarded and commonly used smudge (incense) in Native American ceremonies.

meditation and wake up to our living visions, where scents help us to live more content, relaxed, and stress-free lives. Let us awaken not only to the divinity in nature, but to truly knowing what it means to be more alive (see Photo 6.2).

Appendix A

Resource Directory

Baieido Japanese Incense
http://www.oller.net
An excellent resource on Japanese incense and the Japanese incense ceremony.

Nippon Kodo
http://www.nipponkodo.com/
A leading incense manufacturer in Japan, and one of the best names in Japanese incense. Nippon Kodo is a very old company with a line of high quality products, traditional products, and some natural products.

Organo-Leptic.com
www.Organo-Leptic.com
Experience raw, natural incense by visiting Organo-Leptic.com. Natural incense, as well as other selected natural products, such as raw chocolate, are featured for your sensual enjoyment at this site. Developed by the author of *The Incense Bible,* Kerry Hughes.

Scented Mountain
http://www.scentedmountain.com
Offering the incense of ancient kings and spiritual leaders. Cultivated agarwood is now available for everyone to enjoy.

Scents of Earth
http://www.scentsofearth.com
A very comprehensive incense Web site, offering natural incense of many traditions. This shop is great with customer service and knows its stuff.

Shoyeido Japanese Incense
http://www.shoyeido.com
   Shoyeido is a 300-year-old, traditional Japanese incense company, established in 1705. It produces some of the highest quality incense in the world.

White Lotus Aromatics
http://www.whitelotusaromatics.com/
   A small supplier of high quality essential oils, and a good resource for understanding the high-quality fragrances out of India.

Appendix B

Selected Experts

Andy Baggott
Celtic traditions scholar
Author of *The Celtic Wheel of Life*
E-mail: andy@andybaggott.com
http://www.AndyBaggott.com

Reimar C. Bruening, PhD
Medicinal natural products chemist
E-mail: Rcbruening@mac.com

Chief Phil Crazybull, PhD
Lakota medicine man
Deceased

Krisa Fredrickson, MSc
Ethnobotanist
P.O. Box 6507
Albany, CA 94705-0507
E-mail: krosafredrickson@hotmail.com

Dr. Ira J. Golchehreh, LAC, OMD
Acupuncturist and doctor of Oriental medicine
San Rafael, CA

Constance Grauds, RPh
President, Association of Natural Medicine Pharmacists
Minneapolis, MN
Phone: 612-216-1747
E-mail: anmp@aol.com
http://www.anmp.org

The Incense Bible
© 2007 by The Haworth Press, Inc. All rights reserved.
doi:10.1300/5820_08

Kerry Hughes, MSc
Ethnobotanist and author of *The Incense Bible*
P.O. Box 3222
Vallejo, CA 94590
E-mail: kerry@ethnopharm.com
http://www.ethnopharm.com

Rufino Paxi
Amuta medicine man
Calle Pedro Salazar No. 509
P.O. Box 5442
La Paz, Bolivia

Rev. Thomas Scirghi, SJ
Jesuit School of Theology at Berkeley
Berkeley, California
Phone: 510-549-5032
E-mail: tscirghi@jstb.edu

Rev. Heng Sure, PhD
Senior monastic disciple of the late Chan Master Hsuan Hua
Director of the Berkeley Buddhist Monastery Professor,
Institute For World Religions Assistant Secretary,
Global Council, United Religions Initiative
Berkeley Buddhist Monastery
Berkeley, CA 94703
E-mail: paramita@drba.org

References

Ackerman, D. (1990). *A Natural History of the Senses*. New York: Vintage Books.

Aftel, M. (2001). *Essence and Alchemy: A Book of Perfume*. New York: North Point Press.

Akhondzadeh, S., Kashani, L., Fotouhi, A., Jarvandi, S., Mobaseri, M., Moin, M., Khani, M., Jamshidi, A.H., Baghalian, K., and Taghizadeh, M. (2003). Comparison of *Lavandula angustifolia* Mill. tincture and imipramine in the treatment of mild to moderate depression: A double-blind, randomized trial. *Progress in Neuro-Psychopharmacology & Biological Psychiatry* 27(1):123-127.

Akisue, G. (1969). Pharmacognostic Study of the Balsam and Related Products of Myroxylon-Peruiferum-D. Reports Monographs Non Serials. 151.

Akisue, G. (1972a). Secretions of *Myroxylon peruiferum* Part 2: Physical and chemical characterization of the balsam and qualitative analysis of some components. *Revista De Farmacia E Bioquimica Da Universidade De Sao Paulo* 10(1): 73-96.

Akisue, G. (1972b). Secretions of *Myroxylon peruiferum* Part 3: Physical and chemical characterization of the essential oil of the balsam and qualitative analysis of some components. *Revista De Farmacia E Bioquimica Da Universidade De Sao Paulo* 10(2):151-165.

Atal, C.K. and Kapur, B.M. (Eds.) (1982). *Cultivation and Utilization of Medicinal Plants*. Jammu-Tawi, India: Regional Research Laboratory.

Atchley E.G.C. (1909). *A History of the Use of Incense in Divine Worship*. London: Longmans, Green, and Co.

Bagchi, G.D., Haider, F., Dwivedi, P.D., Singh, S., and Naqvi, A.A. (2003). Effect of different planting dates on the essential oil quality of *Artemisia vulgaris* at northern Indian plain conditions. *Journal of Medicinal & Aromatic Plant Sciences* 25(2):420-423.

Bagi, M.K., Kakrani, H.K., Kalyani, G.A., Satyanarayana, D., and Manvi, F.V. (1985). Preliminary pharmacological studies of essential oil from *Commiphora mukul. Fitoterapia* 56(4):245-248.

Bandoniene, D., Pukalskas, A., Venskutonis, P.R., and Gruzdiene, D. (2000). Preliminary screening of antioxidant activity of some plant extracts in rapeseed oil. *Food Research International* 33(9):785-791.

Barker, S., Grayhem, P., Koon, J., Perkins, J., Whalen, A., and Raudenbush, B. (2003). Improved performance on clerical tasks associated with administration of peppermint odor. *Perceptual and Motor Skills* 97(3) Part 1:1007-1010.

Bartynska, M. and Budzikur-Ramza, E. (2001). The action of some essential oils on fungi. *Bulletin of the Polish Academy of Sciences Biological Sciences* 49(4):327-331.

Bedini, S.A. (1994). *The Trail of Time: Time Measurement with Incense in East Asia.* Cambridge, MA: Cambridge University Press.

Buechele, B., Zugmaier, W., and Simmet, T. (2003). Analysis of pentacyclic triterpenic acids from frankincense gum resins and related phytopharmaceuticals by high-performance liquid chromatography. Identification of lupeolic acid, a novel pentacyclic triterpene. *Journal of Chromatography B* 791(1-2):21-30.

Cardini, F. and Weixin, H. (1998). Moxibustion for correction of breech presentation: A randomized controlled trial. *JAMA: The Journal of the American Medical Association* 280(18):1580-1584.

Case, R.J., Tucker, A.O., Maciarello, M.J., and Wheeler, K.A. (2003). Chemistry and ethnobotany of commercial incense copals, copal blanco, copal oro, and copal negro, of North America. *Economic Botany* 57(2):189-202.

Chen, D. and Haviland-Jones, J. (1999). Rapid mood change and human odors. *Physiology & Behavior* 68(1-2):241-250.

Chomchalow, N. (2001). Utilization of Vetiver as Medicinal and Aromatic Plants: Special Reference to Thailand. Bangkok: Pacific Rim Vetiver Network. Technical Bulletin No. 2001/1, September.

Classen, C., Howes, D., and Synnott, A. (1994). *Aroma: The Cultural History of Smell.* New York: Routledge.

Conelly, W.T. (1985). Copal and rattan collecting in the Philippines. *Economic Botany* 39(1):39-46.

Cornwell, R.E., Boothroyd, L., Burt, D.M., Feinberg, D.R., Jones, B.C., Little, A.C., Pitman, R., Whiten, S., and Perrett, D.I. (2004). Concordant preferences for opposite-sex signals? Human pheromones and facial characteristics. *Proceedings of the Royal Society B: Biological Sciences* 271(1539):635-640.

Cowan, E. (1995). *Plant Spirit Medicine: The Healing Power of Plants.* Columbus, NC: Blue Water Publishing.

DeLeo, V.A., Suarez, S.M., and Maso, M.J. (1992). Photoallergic contact dermatitis. Results of photopatch testing in New York, 1985 to 1990. *Archives of Dermatology* 128(11):1513-1518.

Dentali, S.J. and Hoffmann, J.J. (1992). Potential antiinfective agents from *Eriodictyon angustifolium* and *Salvia apiana. International Journal of Pharmacognosy* 30(3):223-231.

Dodia, S. (2004). In vitro antifungal efficacy of essential oils against keratinophilic fungi isolated from patients of *Tinea capitis. Geobios* (Jodhpur) 31(1):77-78.

Duwiejua, M., Zeitlin, I.J., Waterman, P.G., Chapman, J., Mhango, G.J., and Provan, G.J. (1993). Anti-inflammatory activity of resins from some species of the plant family Burseraceae. *Planta Medica* 59(1):12-16.

Dwivedi, C., Guan, X., Harmsen, W.L., Voss, A.L., Goetz-Parten, D.E., Koopman, E.M., Johnson, K.M., Valluri, H.B., and Matthees, D.P. (2003). Chemopreventive effects of alpha-santalol on skin tumor development in CD-1 and SENCAR mice. *Cancer Epidemiology, Biomarkers & Prevention* 12(2): 151-156.

Edwards, H.G.M. and Moens, L. (2003). Raman spectroscopy of different types of Mexican copal resins. *Spectrochimica Acta,* Part A: Molecular and biomolecular spectroscopy 59A(10).

Eiermann, H.J. (1980). Regulatory issues concerning AETT and 6-MC. *Contact Dermatitis* 6(2):120-122.

Fernandez, X., Lizzani-Cuvelier, L., Loiseau, A.-M., Perichet, C., and Delbecque, C. (2003). Volatile constituents of benzoin gums: Siam and Sumatra. Part 1. *Flavour & Fragrance Journal* 18(4):328-333.

Fischer-Rizzi, S. (1996). *The Complete Incense Book.* New York: Sterling Publishing Company.

Ford, S.L., Steiner, R.R., Thiericke, R., Young, R., and Soine, W.H. (2001). Dragon's blood incense: Misbranded as a drug of abuse? *Forensic Science International* 115(1-2):1-8.

Fraisse, D., Carnat, A., Carnat, A.-P., Guedon, D., and Lamaison, J.-L. (2003). Hydroxycinnamic acid levels of various batches from mugwort flowering tops. *Annales Pharmaceutiques Francaises* 61(4):265-268.

Frey, J. (2003). Pheromones: An underestimated communication signal in humans. *Annales de Biologie Clinique (Paris)* 61(3):275-278.

Friedel, H.D. and Matusch, R. (1987). Isolation and structure elucidation of epimeric 1-5 6 guaiadienes from tolu balsam. *Helvetica Chimica Acta* 70(6):1616-1622.

Galluzzi, L.A. and Kimmerer, R.W. (2003). The basketry plant: *Hierochloe odorata*; sustainable management through indigenous harvesting practices. *Ecological Society of America Annual Meeting Abstracts* 88:117.

Gangrade, S.K., Shrivastava, R.D., Sharma, O.P., Jain, N.K., and Trivedi, K.C. (1991). In-vitro antifungal effect of the essential oils. *Indian Perfumer* 35(1):46-49.

Gangrade, S.K., Shrivastava, R.D., Sharma, O.P., Moghe, M.N., and Trivedi, K.C. (1990). Evaluation of some essential oils for antibacterial properties. *Indian Perfumer* 34(3):204-208.

Garg, S.C. (2000-2001). Ethnomedicine for snake bite. *Journal of Medicinal & Aromatic Plant Sciences* 22-23(4A-1A):546-553.

Gedney, J.J., Glover, T.L., and Fillingim, R.B. (2004). Sensory and affective pain discrimination after inhalation of essential oils. *Psychosomatic Medicine* 66(4): 599-606.

Gonzalez, A.G., Aguiar, Z.E., Grillo, T.A., and Luis, J.G. (1992). Diterpenes and diterpene quinones from the roots of *Salvia apiana*. *Phytochemistry* (Oxford) 31(5):1691-1695.

Gonzalez, A.G., Leon, F., Hernandez, J.C., Padron, J.I., Sanchez-Pinto, L., and Bermejo Barrera, J. (2004). Flavans of dragon's blood from *Dracaena draco* and *Dracaena tamaranae*. *Biochemical Systematics & Ecology* 32(2):179-184.

Hall, D. (1999). *Incense & Thunder.* Sisters, OR: Multnomah Publishers.

Hammer, K.A., Carson, C.F., and Riley, T.V. (1998). In-vitro activity of essential oils, in particular *Melaleuca alternifolia* (tea tree) oil and tea tree soil products, against *Candida* spp. *Journal of Antimicrobial Chemotherapy* 42(5):591-595.

Hayakawa, R., Matsunaga, K., and Arima, Y. (1987). Depigmented contact dermatitis due to incense. *Contact Dermatitis* 16(5):272-274.

Himmelreich, U., Masaoud, M., Adam, G., and Ripperger, H. (1995). Damalachawin, a triflavonoid of new structural type from dragon's blood of *Dracaena cinnabari*. *Phytochemistry* (Oxford) 39(4):949-951.

Howes, M.-J.R., Simmonds, M.S.J., and Kite, G.C. (2004). Evaluation of the quality of sandalwood essential oils by gas chromatography-mass spectrometry. *Journal of Chromatography A* 1028(2):307-312.

Hwang, Y.-S., Wu, K.-H., Kumamoto, J., Axelrod, H., and Mulla, M.S. (1985). Isolation and identification of mosquito repellents in *Artemisia vulgaris*. *Journal of Chemical Ecology* 11(9):1297-1306.

Hyams, G. (2004). *Incense: Rituals, Mystery, Lore.* San Francisco: Chronicle Books.

Ishihara, M., Masatsugu, Y., and Uneyama, K. (1992). Preparation of (levo)-guaia-1(10),11-dien-15,2-olide and (levo)-2-alpha-hydroxyguaia-1(10),11-dien-15-oic acid, fragrant sesquiterpenes in agarwood (*Aquilaria agallocha* Roxb.). *Tetrahedron* 48(47):10265-10276.

Ishihara, M., Tsuneya, T., Shiga, M., and Uneyama, K. (1991). Three sesquiterpenes from agarwood. *Phytochemistry* (Oxford) 30(2):563-566.

Ishihara, M., Tsuneya, T., and Uneyama, K. (1991). Guaiane sesquiterpenes from agarwood. *Phytochemistry* (Oxford) 30(10):3343-3348.

Ishihara, M., Tsuneya, T., and Uneyama, K. (1993). Fragrant sesquiterpenes from agarwood. *Phytochemistry* (Oxford) 33(5):1147-1155.

Jerkovic, I., Mastelic, J., Milos, M., Juteau, F., Masotti, V., and Viano, J. (2003). Chemical variability of *Artemisia vulgaris* L. essential oils originated from the Mediterranean area of France and Croatia. *Flavour & Fragrance Journal* 18(5): 436-440.

Jiang, D.-F., Ma, P., Wang, X.-H., Zhang, L.-Q., Li, Q.-D., Wang, J.-L., Cheng, Z.-Y., and Yang, C.-R. (1995). The studies of fungal population and relationship between fungi and forming of dragon's blood resin in *Dracaena cochinchinensis*. *Acta Botanica Yunnanica* 17(1):79-82.

Jirovetz, L., Buchbauer, G., Jaeger, W., Woidich, A., and Nikiforov, A. (1992). Analysis of fragrance compounds in blood samples of mice by gas chromatography mass spectrometry GC-FTIR and GC-AES after inhalation of sandalwood oil. *Biomedical Chromatography* 6(3):133-134.

Johnson, P. (Trans.). (1998). *Medicine of the Prophet.* Cambridge, UK: The Islamic Texts Society.

Kakrani, H.K. and Kalyani, G.A. (1984). Antihelminthic activity of essential oil of *Commiphora mukul*. *Fitoterapia* 55(4):232-234.

Kasali, A.A., Adio, A.M., Oyedeji, A.O., Eshilokun, A.O., and Adefenwa, M. (2002). Volatile constituents of *Boswellia serrata* Roxb. (Burseraceae) bark. *Flavour & Fragrance Journal* 17(6):462-464.

Kashio, M. and Johnson, D. (2001). Monograph on Benzoin (Balsamic Resin from Sytrax Species). Bangkok: Food and Agriculture Organization of the United Nations.

Kim, Y.C., Lee, E.H., Lee, Y.M., Kim, H.K., Song, B.K., Lee, E.J., and Kim, H.M. (1997). Effect of the aqueous extract of *Aquilaria agallocha* stems on the immediate hypersensitivity reactions. *Journal of Ethnopharmacology* 58(1):31-38.

Kimmatkar, N., Thawani, V., Hingorani, L., and Khiyani, R. (2003). Efficacy and tolerability of *Boswellia serrata* extract in treatment of osteoarthritis of knee: A randomized double blind placebo controlled trial. *Phytomedicine* (Jena) 10(1):3-7.

Knight, L., Levin, A., and Mendenhall, C. (2001). Candles and Incense as Potential Sources of Indoor Air Pollution: Market Analysis and Literature Review. January; EPA Contract 68-D7-0001 Washington, D.C.: U.S. Environmental Protection Agency, Office of Research and Development. http://www.epa.gov/ordntrnt/ORD/NRMRL/Publications/329600R01001.htm.

Konishi, T., Konoshima, T., Shimada, Y., and Kiyosawa, S. (2002). Six new 2-(2-phenylethyl) chromones from agarwood. *Chemical & Pharmaceutical Bulletin* (Tokyo) 50(3):419-422.

Langenheim, J.H. (2004). *Plant Resins: Chemistry, Evolution, Ecology, Ethnobotany.* Portland, OR: Timber Press.

Larsen, W.G. (1985). Perfume dermatitis. *Journal of the American Academy of Dermatology* 12(1) Part 1:1-9.

Lee, S.-J., Chung, H.-Y., Maier, C.G.-A., Wood, A.R., Dixon, R.A., and Mabry, T.J. (1998). Estrogenic flavonoids from *Artemisia vulgaris* L. *Journal of Agricultural & Food Chemistry* 46(8):3325-3329.

Linares E. and Bye R.A. Jr. (1987). A study of four medicinal plant complexes of Mexico and adjacent USA. *Journal of Ethnopharmacology* 19(2):153-184.

Luo, M., Fee, M.S., and Katz L.C. (2003). Encoding pheromonal signals in the accessory olfactory bulb of behaving mice. *Science* 299(5610):1196-1201.

Mabberley, D.J. (1997). *The Plant-Book: A Portable Dictionary of the Vascular Plants,* Second Edition. Cambridge, UK: Cambridge University Press.

Maranduba, A., De Oliveira, A.B., De Oliveira, G.G., Reis, J.E.D.P., and Gottlieb, O.R. (1979). Iso flavonoids from *Myroxylon peruiferum. Phytochemistry* (Oxford) 18(5):815-818.

Masago, R., Matsuda, T., Kikuchi, Y., Miyazaki, Y., Iwanaga, K., Harada, H., and Katsuura, T. (2000). Effects of inhalation of essential oils on EEG activity and sensory evaluation. *Journal of Physiological Anthropology & Applied Human Science* 19(1): 35-42.

Masaoud, M., Himmelreich, U., Ripperger, H., and Adam, G. (1995). New biflavonoids from dragon's blood of *Dracaena cinnabari. Planta Medica* 61(4): 341-344.

Masaoud, M., Ripperger, H., Himmelreich, U., and Adam, G. (1995). Cinnabarone, a biflavonoid from dragon's blood of *Dracaena cinnabari*. *Phytochemistry* (Oxford) 38(3):751-753.

Masaoud, M., Ripperger, H., Porzel, A., and Adam, G. (1995). Flavonoids of dragon's blood from *Dracaena cinnabari*. *Phytochemistry* (Oxford) 38(3):745-749.

Masaoud, M., Schmidt, J., and Adam, G. (1995). Sterols and triterpenoids from *Dracaena cinnabari*. *Phytochemistry* (Oxford) 38(3):795-796.

McCampbell, H. (2002). *Sacred Smoke: The Ancient Art of Smudging for Modern Times*. Summertown, TN: Native Voices.

McMahone, C. (2001) Incense in India: Visit to Myosore and the story of incense.White Lotus Aromatics Newsletter—Issue: Incense, August 30, 2001 Available at http://www.whitelotusaromatics.com/newsletters/incense.html.

Methacanon, P., Chaikumpollert, O., Thavorniti, P., and Suchiva, K. (2003). Hemicellulosic polymer from vetiver grass and its physicochemical properties. *Carbohydrate Polymers* 54(3):335-342.

Michaelis, K., Vostrowsky, O., Paulini, H., Zintl, R., and Knobloch, K. (1982). Essential oil components from blossom of *Artemisia vulgaris*. *Zeitschrift fur Naturforschung* 37(3-4):152-158.

Monard, A. and Grenier, A. (1969). Study of balsam of Peru of various origins by means of thin layer and gas phase chromatography. In De Moerloose, P. (Chairman), *Fifth International Symposium on Chromatography and Electrophoresis* (pp. 529-540). Ann Arbor, MI: Humphrey Science Publishers, Inc.

Moore, M. (1993). *Medicinal Plants of the Pacific West*. Santa Fe, NM: Red Crane Books.

Morita, K. (1992). *The Book of Incense*. Tokyo: Kodansha International.

Morton, J.F. (1981). *Atlas of Medicinal Plants of Middle America. Bahamas to Yucatan*. Springfield, IL: C.C. Thomas.

Moss, M., Cook, J., Wesnes, K., and Duckett, P. (2003). Aromas of rosemary and lavender essential oils differentially affect cognition and mood in healthy adults. *The International Journal of Neuroscience* 113(1):15-38.

Müller-Ebeling, C, Ratsch, C., and Bahadur Shahi, S. (2000). *Shamanism and Tantra in the Himalayas*. Rochester, VT: Inner Traditions.

Naef, R., Velluz, A., Brauchli, R., and Thommen, W. (1995). Agarwood oil (*Aquilaria agallocha* Roxb.): Its composition and eight new valencane-, eremophilane- and vetispirane-derivatives. *Flavour & Fragrance Journal* 10(3):147-152.

Naef, R., Velluz, A., Busset, N., and Gaudin, J.-M. (1992). New nor-sesquiterpenoids with 10-epieudesmane skeleton from agarwood (*Aquilaria agallocha* Roxb.). *Flavour & Fragrance Journal* 7(6):295-298.

Nakamura, N., Kiuchi, F., Tsuda, Y., Kondo, K., and Sato, T. (1990). Nematocidal and bursting activities of essential oils on the larvae of *Toxocara canis*. *Shoyakugaku Zasshi* 44(3):183-195.

Nitta, A., Tani, S., Sakamaki, E., and Saito, Y. (1984). On the source and evaluation of benzoin. *Yakugaku Zasshi* 104(6):592-600.

Okugawa, H., Ueda, R., Matsumoto, K., Kawanishi, K., and Kato, A. (1993). Effects of agarwood extracts on the central nervous system in mice. *Planta Medica* 59(1):32-36.

Okugawa, H., Ueda, R., Matsumoto, K., Kawanishi, K., and Kato, A. (1996). Effect of Jinkoh-eremol and agarospirol from agarwood on the central nervous system in mice. *Planta Medica* 62(1):2-6.

Park, M.K. and Lee, E.S. (2004). The effect of aroma inhalation method on stress responses of nursing students. *Taehan Kanho Hakhoe Chi* 34(2):344-351.

Pastorova, I., De Koster, C.G., and Boon, J.J. (1997). Analytical study of free and ester bound benzoic and cinnamic acids of gum benzoin resins by GC-MS and HPLC-frit FAB-MS. *Phytochemical Analysis* 8(2):63-73.

Pattnaik, S., Subramanyam, V.R., and Kole, C. (1996). Antibacterial and antifungal activity of ten essential oils in vitro. *Microbios* 86(349):237-245.

Pearson, J. and Prendergast, H.D.V. (2001). *Daemonorops, Dracaena* and other dragon's blood. *Economic Botany* 55(4):474-477.

Pignatti, E.W. (1979). The presence of *Hierochloe odorata* in Italy. *Giornale Botanico Italiano* 113(1-2):69-74.

Pukalskas, A., Van Beek, T.A., Venskutonis, R.P., Linssen, J.P.H., van Veldhuizen, A., and de Groot, A. (2002). Identification of radical scavengers in sweet grass (*Hierochloe odorata*). *Journal of Agricultural & Food Chemistry* 50(10):2914-2919.

Pungle, P., Banavalikar, M., Suthar, A., Biyani, M., and Mengi, S. (2003). Immunomodulatory activity of boswellic acids of *Boswellia serrata* Roxb. *Indian Journal of Experimental Biology* 41(12):1460-1462.

Quezada, R.S. (2003). Therapeutic oil composition. *Official Gazette of the United States Patent & Trademark Office Patents* 1271(4). Patent number 6582736. Available at: http://www.patentstorm.us/patents/6582736-fulltext.html.

Rai, S.N. (1981). Regional volume tables for Indian copal *Vateria indica* tree and its certain other relationships data from Karnataka India. *Indian Journal of Forestry* 4(2):99-102.

Rai, S.N. and Sarma, C.R. (1990). Depleting sandalwood production and rising prices. *Indian Forester* 116(5):348-355.

Ramachandran, V.S. (1999). *Phantoms in the Brain: Probing the Mysteries of the Human Mind.* New York: Perennial.

Reichling, J., Schmoekel, H., Fitzi, J., Bucher, S., and Saller, R. (2004). Dietary support with *Boswellia* resin in canine inflammatory joint and spinal disease. *Schweizer Archiv Fuer Tierheilkunde* 146(2):71-80.

Sangat-Roemantyo, H. (1990). Ethnobotany of the Javanese Indonesia incense. *Economic Botany* 44(3):413-416.

Saxena, V.K. and Sharma, R.N. (1998). Constituents of the essential oil from *Commiphora mukul* gum resin. *Journal of Medicinal & Aromatic Plant Sciences* 20(1):55-56.

Scala, A., Overton, S., Zitka, M., and Ryan, D. (2001). Antifungal activities of two essential oils in the prevention of mildew infection (*Blumeris graminis*) in wheat (*Triticum* spp.). *Phytopathology* 91(6 Supplement):S197.

Serrano, H. and Garcia-Suarez, M.D. (2001). Sperm aggregation by water extracts from two *Bursera* species. *Archives of Andrology* 46(1):15-20.

Shimada, Y. and Kiyosawa, S. (1984). Studies on the agarwood jinko 3. The histochemical study of the resinoid tissues. *Shoyakugaku Zasshi* 38(4): 321-326.

Shin, S. (2003). Anti-*Aspergillus* activities of plant essential oils and their combination effects with ketoconazole or amphotericin B. *Archives of Pharmacal Research* (Seoul) 26(5);389-393.

Silvotti, L., Montani, G., and Tirindelli, R. (2003). How mammals detect pheromones. *Journal of Endocrinological Investigation* 26(3 Suppl):49-53.

Singh, R.P., Singh, R., Ram, P., and Batliwala, P.G. (1993). Use of pushkar-guggul, an indigenous antiischemic combination, in the management of ischemic heart disease. *International Journal of Pharmacognosy* 31(2):147-160.

Soehartono, T. and Newton, A. (2002). The Gaharu trade in Indonesia: Is it sustainable? *Economic Botany* 56(3):271-284.

Spencer, P.S., Sterman, A.B., Horoupian, D.S., and Foulds, M.M. (1979). Neurotoxic fragrance produces ceroid and myelin disease. *Science* 204(4393):633-635.

Stross, B. (1997). Mesoamerican copal resins. *U Mut Maya* 6:177-186. Available at: http://www.blackwell-synergy.com/doi/abs/10.1111/j.1475-4754.2006.00259.x?cookieSet=1&journalCode=arch.

Sutton, A. (2000). The spiritual significance of the Qetoret: The inner meaning of incense. Available at http://www.oller.net/qetoret.htm.

Tezuka, T., Kusuda, S., Higashida, T., Matsumura, H., Horikawa, T., and Tamaki, A. (1993). The clinical effects of mugwort extract on pruritic skin lesions. *Skin Research* 35(2):303-311.

Thorne, F., Neave, N., Scholey, A., Moss, M., and Fink, B. (2002). Effects of putative male pheromones on female ratings of male attractiveness: Influence of oral contraceptives and the menstrual cycle. *Neuro Endocrinology Letters* 23(4):291-297.

Tripitaka Master Shikshananda of Khotan (trans. to Chinese). Dharma Realm Buddhist University (trans. to English). (1981) Flower Adornment Sutra. Chapter 39, Part IV. Entering the Dharma Realm. Talmage, California.

Trotter, K., Dallas, K., and Verdone, P. (1988). Olfactory stimuli and their effects on REM dreams. *Psychiatric Journal of the University of Ottawa [Revue de Psychiatrie de l'Université d'Ottawa]* 13(2):94-96.

Tucker, A.O. (1986). Frankincense and myrrh. *Economic Botany* 40(4):425-433.

Vachalkova, A., Novotny, L., Nejedlikova, M., and Suchy, V. (1995). Potential carcinogenicity of homoisoflavanoids and flavonoids from *Resina sanguinis draconis* (*Dracaena cinnabari* Balf.). *Neoplasma* (Bratislava) 42(6):313-316.

Venkataramanan, M.N., Borthakur, R., and Singh, H.D. (1985). Occurrence of endotrophic mycorrhizal fungus in agarwood plant *Aquillaria agallocha. Current Science* (Bangalore) 54(18):928.

Voeks, R. (1997). *The Sacred Leaves of Candomble: African Magic, Medicine, and Religion in Brazil.* Austin: University of Texas Press.

Wahlberg, I. and Enzell, C.R. (1971). 3 oxo-6beta-hydroxy olean-12-en-28-oic-acid a new tri terpenoid from commercial tolu balsam. *Acta Chemica Scandinavica* 25(1):70-76.

Wahlberg, I., Hjelte, M.B., Karlsson, K., and Enzell, C.R. (1971). Constituents of commercial tolu balsam. *Acta Chemica Scandinavica* 25(9):3285-3295.

Wang, J.-L., Li, X.-C., Jiang, D.-F., Ma, P., and Yang, C.-R. (1995). Chemical constituents of dragon's blood resin from *Dracaena cochinchinensis* in Yunnan and their antifungal activity. *Acta Botanica Yunnanica* 17(3):336-340.

Wang, X., Greilberger, J., Ledinski, G., Kager, G., Paigen, B., and Jurgens, G. (2004). The hypolipidemic natural product *Commiphora mukul* and its component guggulsterone inhibit oxidative modification of LDL. *Atherosclerosis* 172(2):239-246.

Watt, J.M. and Breyer-Brandwijk, M.G. (1962). The *Medicinal and Poisonous Plants of Southern and Eastern Africa,* Second Edition. London: E. & S. Livingstone, Ltd.

Williams, R.M. (2004). Fragrance alters mood and brain chemistry—Health risks and environmental issues. *Townsend Letter For Doctors & Patients* (April).

Wohrl, S., Hemmer, W., Focke, M., Gotz, M., and Jarisch, R. (2001). The significance of fragrance mix, balsam of Peru, colophony and propolis as screening tools in the detection of fragrance allergy. *British Journal of Dermatology* 145(2):268-273.

Wysocki, C.J., Nyby, J., Whitney, G., Beauchamp, G.K., and Katz, Y. (1982). The vomeronasal organ: primary role in mouse chemosensory gender recognition. *Physiology & Behavior* 29(2):315-327.

Yamagata, E and Yoneda, K. (1986a). Pharmacognostic studies on the crude drug of agarwood III. Differentiation of agarwood by discriminant analysis. *Shoyakugaku Zasshi* 40(3):266-270.

Yamagata, E. and Yoneda, K. (1986b). Pharmacognostic studies on the crude drug of agarwood V. Evaluation of agarwood by principal component analysis and factor analysis. *Shoyakugaku Zasshi* 40(3):275-280.

Yamagata, E. and Yoneda, K. (1987). Pharmacognostical studies on the crude drug of agarwood VI. On Kanankoh. *Shoyakugaku Zasshi* 41(2):142-146.

Yoneda, K. et al. (1984). Sesquiterpenoids in two different kinds of agarwood. *Phytochemistry* 23(9):2068-2069.

Yoneda, K., Yamagata, E., and Mizuno, M. (1986). Pharmacognostic studies on the crude drug of agarwood II. On the Chinese agarwood. *Shoyakugaku Zasshi* 40(3):259-265.

Yoneda, K., Yamagata, E., Sugimoto, Y., and Nakanishi, T. (1986). Pharmacognostic studies on the crude drug of agarwood I. Comparison of the constituents of the essential oil from agarwood by means of GLC and GC-MS. *Shoyakugaku Zasshi* 40(3):252-258.

Yu, J.G., Cong, P.Z., Lin, J.T., and Fang, H.J. (1988). Studies on the chemical constituents of Chinese sandalwood oil and preliminary structures of five novel compounds. *Yaoxue Xuebao* 23(11):868-872.

Zhou Z.-H., Wang, J.-L., and Yang, C.-R. (2001). Cochinchinenin: A new chalcone dimer from the Chinese dragon blood. *Yaoxue Xuebao* 36(3):200-204.

Zhu, N., Sheng, S., Sang, S., Rosen, R.T., and Ho, C.-T. (2003). Isolation and characterization of several aromatic sesquiterpenes from *Commiphora myrrha*. *Flavour & Fragrance Journal* 18(4):282-285.

Index

Page numbers followed by the letter "p" indicate photos; those followed by the letter "t" indicate tables.

Vietnamese New Year, 174
Vision of incense use, 15, 163-165
Vision Quest, 83, 164
Voeks, Robert, 91
Voice quality and frankincense, 122
Vomeronasal organ, 30
Voodoo, 91

Walk in beauty, 169-170
Wamira of Papua New Guinea, 33
Water, incense, 67-68
Water clock, 51, 52
"Way of the thunderbolt," 73
The Way of Incense (Koh-do), 12, 13,
   74-76
Weddings, 64, 174
Weight loss and peppermint essential
   oil, 49-50
Wheel of Luminosity, 163
White Buffalo Calf Woman, 85
White sage
   California white sage, 178p
   chemical constituents, 141
   description of plant, 139
   Native American medicine, 85-86
   overview, 138-139
   smudge, 139, 140

White sage *(continued)*
   smudge stick, 146-147, 147p
   usage, 139-141
Whores, smell of, 27-28
Witch doctor, 7
Witchcraft, 29, 54, 171-172
Women as frivolous creatures, 26-27, 28
Wood incense, 146
Workout trends, 6-7
Worldwide ritual, 1, 3-4
Worship. *See also* Religion
   for Christians, 80
   Eucharistic liturgy, 80-82
   incense usage, 176-177
   Indian Hindu worship, 63-65
   Japanese Buddhism, 69-70
Wu, Emperor, 66

Yagna, 63
Yemen, production of frankincense and
   myrrh, 60
Yew, 88
Yoga, 6-7, 163

Zen in Japan, 68
Zeus, 20

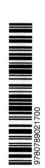